Retreat Recipes for Yoga Lovers

by Debra Mazer

Welcome!

In these shifting times, birthing times, birthing to our intentions + desires, we have the capacity to reclaim our sovereignty + health. Ritual helps. Creating your own food at home, using locally grown ingredients, is so healing, soothing + grounding. Create a routine for yourself. Let it be your practice. Your healing. Your self-care. Your nurturing. Now is the time. OUR time. To Rise! **You are so worth it. We need you. And you deserve this!**

Enjoy!

With Love + Blessings,

xo Debra.

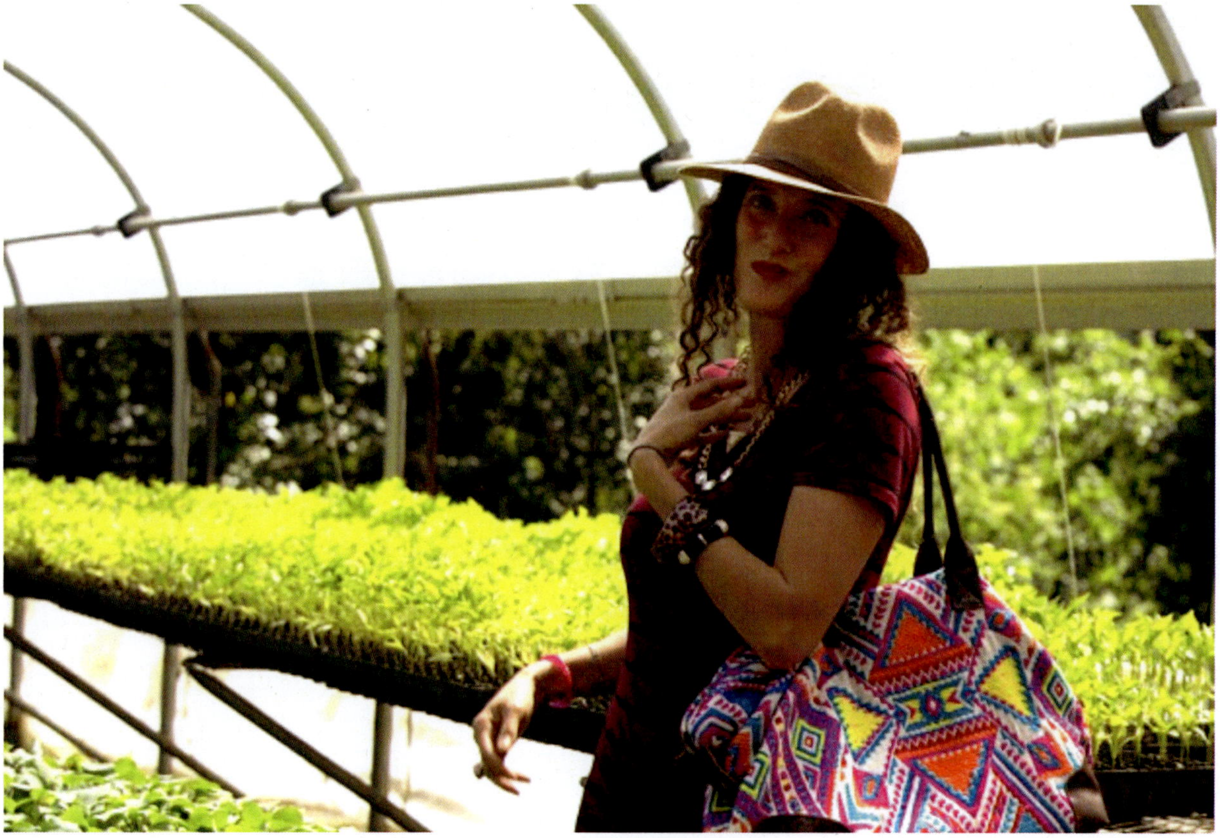

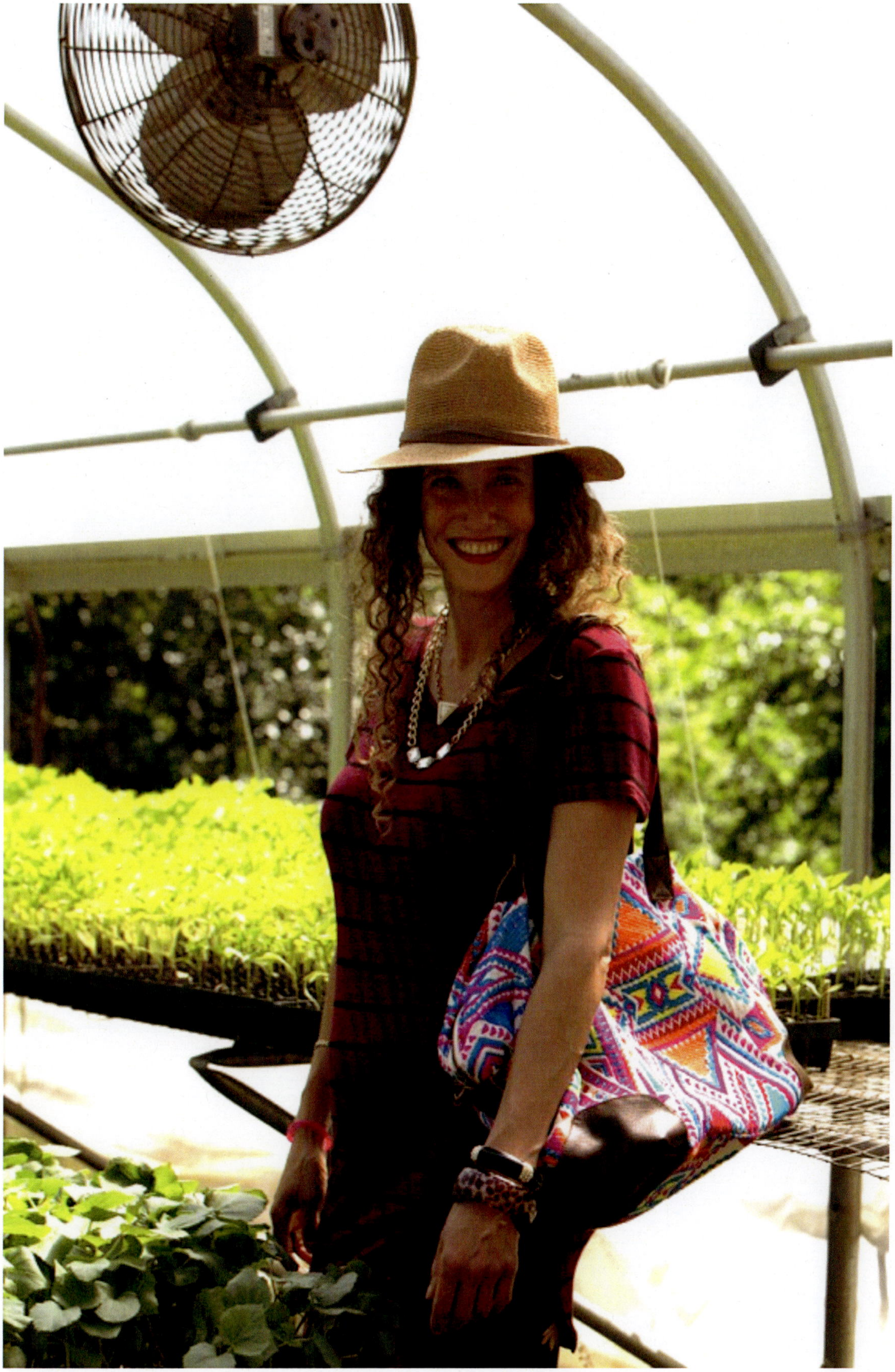

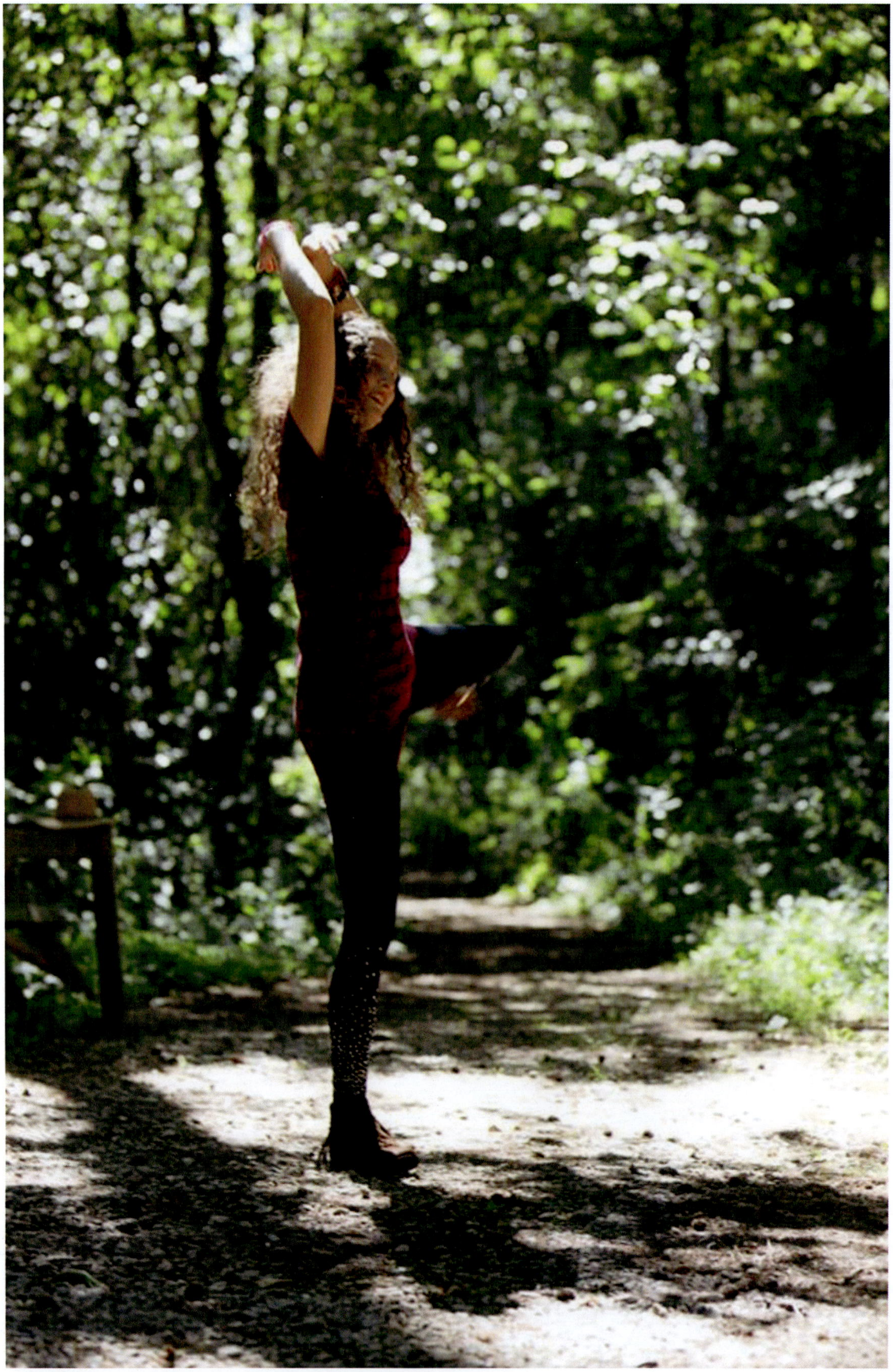

Art/ Photo Credits:

Recipe Lettering Art by Debra Mazer + Kitchen Goddesses

All Photos of Debra (beginning + end) are by AnaRosePhotography.com
All Other Photos are by Debra Mazer

Integrity: Thank you for purchasing this book! Please do not share or reproduce in any way, any portion of this book. This includes photocopy, email, uploading/ or downloading with the intent of sharing. Let's support independent artists + keep good karma circulating for all. Failure to do so will result in legal action. To become an affiliate of Retreat Recipes for Yoga Lovers, visit DebraMazer.com.

A Medical Note: Although I am a Holistic Health Coach + Award-Winning Chef, I am not a Medical Doctor. Particularly if you do have health concerns, and are ready to shift your food/ lifestyle: Please tune into your intuition, grounded self-care + common sense, and see a Doctor/ Wellness Practitioner of your choice. This book is not a substitute for Medical Advice. Please care for yourself, in all ways.

And Another Disclaimer: Mention of companies, websites, and authorities does not imply that they endorse this book. However, we hope they do! ;) Likewise, mention of companies, websites, and authorities does not imply that they are endorsed by Debra Mazer/ Debra Mazer Enterprises LLC. These companies are mentioned as a service to you! I do not receive affiliate commissions for any of them, except for **Institute for Integrative Nutrition**, where I am a proud Graduate + Ambassador. ;)

Please send Fan Mail, Fan Gifts + Packages, Other Delightful Surprises to:

Debra Mazer
P.O. Box 92841
Long Beach, CA 90809

Also, for more Love, please visit:

DebraMazer.com

Table of Contents:

But first, story time…

My Background: When Shiva Rea contacted me to cater a Yoga Retreat on Chumash land in Malibu a year + a half ago, she was clear the food needed to be Gluten-Free, Soy-Free, + Sugar-Free. Add Vegetarian, Mostly Vegan, Seasonal, Local + Organic! This sounded like a match made in Heaven for me, as I call myself a "Debratarian" + my personal food choices much reflect this!

I've been a Raw Food Chef since 2002 professionally, worked in Raw Cafes, as an Instructor at The Living Foods Institute in Atlanta, Personal Chef, private caterer for a dinner honoring Kris Carr, Kitchen Staff for David Wolfe Retreats in Hawaii, + so much more!

While living in Atlanta, I hosted 4-Course Raw Dinner Parties on the Full Moon, + later operated a Weekly Raw Food Delivery Service, called Vibrance, which magnetized its own fame on the covers of the Atlanta Journal-Constitution!

Meanwhile, my own diet was shifting, from 100% Raw, to incorporating Cooked Food again. I enrolled in the Institute for Integrative Nutrition in 2011, + this program changed my life! Gone were the labels + boxing myself in. I gave myself permission to experiment with free-range local eggs + raw cheese. I went to the store + bought organic brown rice to cook, for the first time in many, many years of "Raw" aspiring.

The fascinating part is that the "Food Faeries" did not abandon me, in my transition from being an Award-Winning Raw Chef, to incorporating Cooked Foods (in big pots + pans, to boot!). Just the same way that the spices would speak to me, telling me how much to add + what to change, like a painter painting a canvas, I still receive this "download from Spirit" while cooking these foods.

Some say, "Food is My Gift." Yet, I say, when you are open, when you have a daily practice, when you do The Artist's Way + meditate, + pray, + journal, + do yoga, + whatever your practice, Spirit begins speaking through you. As it has done through me, food being just one of my artistic mediums. I am also a writer, a dancer, a singer in the Agape Choir, + an Intuitive Life, Business, + Holistic Health Coach!

Spirit speaks through me every day, + I know it speaks through you too! Listen, + surrender to your calling. Paint the colors you are asked to paint, + surrender to the experience!

Cooking isn't all about recipes to me. It actually took some discipline to stop + write this all down, because usually it is just me + my blender, or pots + pans, seeing what I have, what's in season, + going from there. I learned how to make food on ecovillages + farms, + it was all about using what we grew + what was available.

I invite you to play with these recipes, change them, add to them, use them as inspiration for yourselves!

You can also follow them exactly, + I promise you a wonderful, exciting learning about Gluten-Free, Vegetarian + Vegan Foods!

An Updated Prayer…

Bag Lady: Besides being one of the best songs by Erykah Badu, this book contains photos of bags from my collection (yes, not just food!) You'll see bags on the cover pages too. Bags for me symbolize openness to collection. Learning, growth, absorption. Adventure, travel, mementos. These recipes have been collected over the course of 16+ years. They have been inspired by various travels. Some of them are recipes that are inspired by another food creatress, who has given me permission to share my version of their recipe in this book.

I love bags. What can I say? I hope you enjoy my illustration quirks! xoxox

Design + Solar Eclipse 2017: This book traveled to Bali. It began in Summer of 2016, as I photographed recipes from my collection at Shiva Rea Retreats in Malibu, California. I spent months working on it every day, promising to do a recipe a day, sitting at cafes, checking in with my writing friends, and just doing it! Fear is most of the battle. And then, it's about discipline + time. (I'm happy to be your Life Coach if you want to write a book! ;))

The evening before the Solar Eclipse, August 2017, this book was born. I stayed up until 5am, + completely transformed the photos. This book is infused with energy. The energy of wealth + healing + love. I hope you will feel its high vibrations + that it uplifts your life, + brings you into greater health, happiness, + wellness. And So It Is. Ashe. Amen. + Blessed Be.

Black Lives Matter + Cultural Diversity: It goes without saying, but I'm going to say it anyway. I transformed this book to include more images of dear ones of color. I believe changing the media changes the world. This book is specifically infused with the intention to honor cultural diversity, harmony + peace. I hold a vision for the Beloved Community. I am by no means an expert on various cultural foods, but simply inspired to share a message of diversity + culture. My own heritage is Jewish, born + raised in the United States. May this book be a blessing to the world. May it uplift humanity. Ashe. Amen. And Blessed Be. Hallelujah!!!

Affirmative Prayer: I am so Grateful for this moment, this Day. I am grateful for you, Reader, that you are here drinking up this Juicy, beautiful book! I am so grateful for the chance to create my Art, + make a living from it! I am so grateful we are here together, co-creating the world we want to see.

I know there is One Power in the Universe, God/ Goddess, Creator/ Spirit, Eternal Higher Self/ Higher Truth. Love + Oneness. The whole of humanity. The cycle of life. Beauty, Wholeness, + Love.

I know I am one with this Power + so are You. I am one with the absolute Wellness of all creation, the Wholeness, Creativity + Peace. It is always flowing through me, as my life, my existence. As this is true for me, I know it is true for you. You are always Protected + Guided by the Divine.

Knowing this, I bless your journey. I bless your journey with Food + Life. I bless you on your Unfolding. I bless us all. May we each be here, to be who we came here to be! Knowing that Life needs us. Each + every one of us. May the path be smooth + full of flow, synchronicities, love, friendship, + laughter.

And may we all have what we need, at all times, in all ways.

I am so Grateful + Thankful to know this Truth. To have the opportunity to pray with you together.

And I release this prayer into the Universe, knowing it is multiplied abundantly!

And So It Is. Amen. *(Yes, I am an Agape Certified Prayer Warrior! I love to mix spirituality with food! ;))*

Debra's organic cuisine is an extraordinary experience of nutritional ecstasy, whether for a catered meal or a Hot Love [Chocolate] Truffle - this is passionate, life-giving food!" – **Shiva Rea**

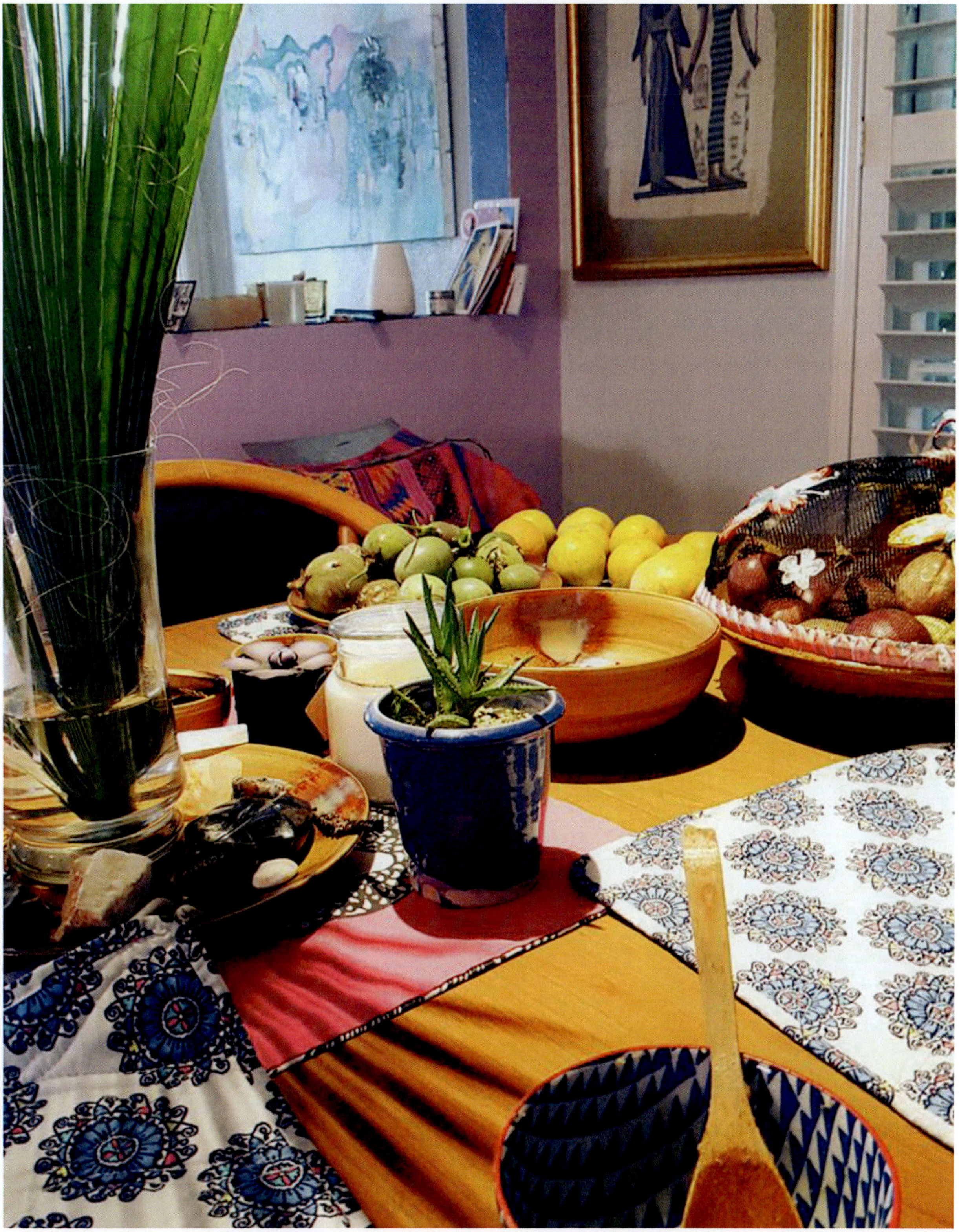

What It's Like to Cater for Shiva Rea: Many of these recipes were created during a year of catering for Shiva Rea's Yoga Retreats. What an amazing experience this has been! One of my favorite things about Shiva Rea is that she is a conscious white woman around race + diverse culture. I also love that she is a "faerie": delightful in her teachings, + also in my communications with her! She stays in the light + consciously infuses with love, her words, energy, + mark on the planet! I can feel it, even in our emails! Thank You Shiva for this amazing opportunity to work with you. I also ***adore*** all of the amazing, high-vibrational yoga lovers Shiva attracts. It has been my pleasure to serve such grateful, enlightened beings! And to be in the energy of retreat, yoga, + healing, is a dream!

How to be a Leader/ Facilitate a Collective: Whew! There are so many Leadership Lessons to be learned, in cooking for a huge event, + managing a Kitchen Crew! From interviewing + hiring, to Group Introductions, Contracts, intention-setting, rules + schedules, there is soooo much involved in catering an event, that most people wouldn't know! ;) I drove around listening to leadership tapes in my car, + I am still a work in progress. It helped that my Sociology/ Women's Studies undergraduate thesis was all about facilitating collectives + bringing diverse people together. What an adventure! Working/ living together, for hours a day, for days upon end, while also sharing a bathroom + room! It is the stuff that deep, lasting friendships + sisterhood are made of, + I am Grateful to each + every one of you, for your intensely hard work, chopping, mixing, blending, stirring, smiling, greeting, + loving. I am also grateful for our relationships! Something happens when you share intensive live-in experiences with others. It's kind of like overnight camp, except more opportunities for conflict + pushing each other's buttons can happen.

It helps to do daily check-ins, to offer a space of clear, open communication, even + especially when it's hard. Because ultimately, our love + harmony goes into the food, into each other, into Life!

I love you. I love you all. Thank You for helping me grow + become a better leader, + not just a vegetable whisperer! ;)

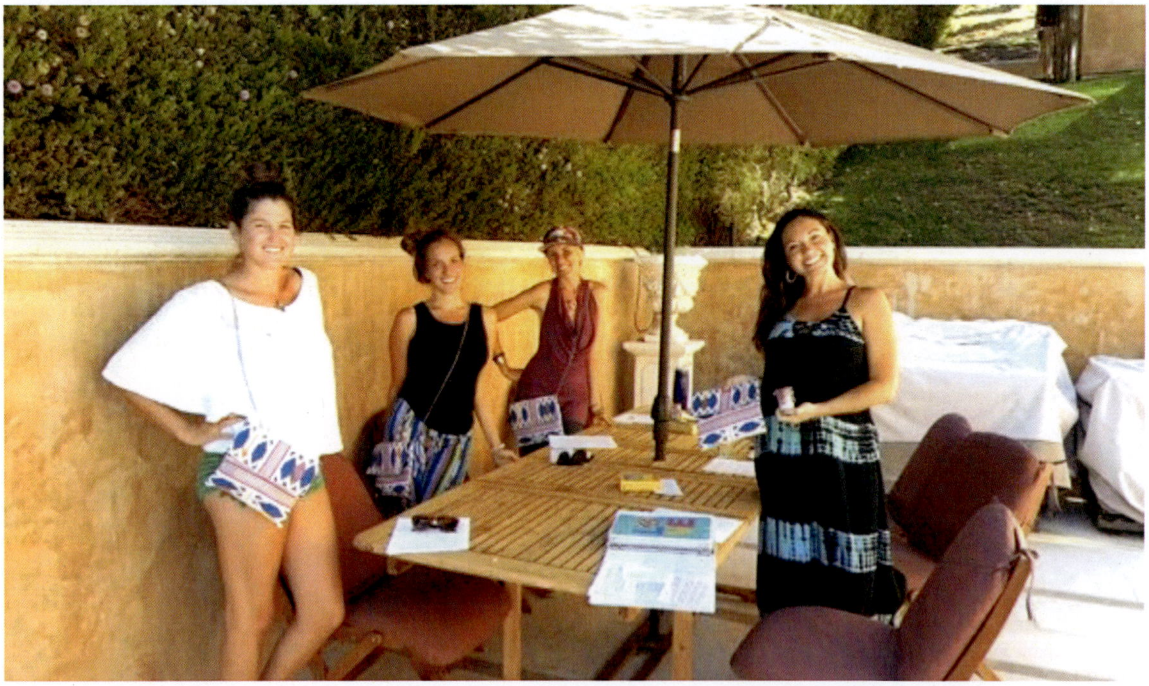

Gratitude

Shout-Out to my Inspirations: First, a shout-out to my Inspirations. For this book: Vegan Richa, Afya Ibomu, Minimalist Baker, Nirvana Cakery, Veg Recipes of India, Café Gratitude. You gave me ideas about cooking from around the world, + opened my mind to new ideas!

Blasts from the past: a thank you to Jackie Graff, whose raw kitchen I first volunteered in, in 2001. I was amazed that you could make nut cheese in a blender! Thank You, Jackie, for your legacy, + for being my "Mother-in-Raw" along with Gideon, my "Father-in-Raw!" Jackie, you are my ultimate Raw Food Teacher. Thank You. I'd also like to give a shout-out to Lov'n It Live, one of the best, most interesting Raw Food Restaurants in Atlanta. Jamaican Patties that are Vegan + Raw?! I say, YES! Thank You to Everlasting Life for giving me my first job as a Raw Chef.

Thank You to The Living Foods Institute, for both changing my world, + then bringing me into your world, as Kitchen Director for 2 years! Another Gratitude for Terces + Matthew Engelhart, my Vegetarian Restaurant heroes, whose books + workshops on communication + business have also altered my life for the better. Thank You to Dancing Rabbit Ecovillage, Twin Oaks Community, + The Local Farmstand in Atlanta, Georgia for teaching me so much about local, seasonal foods. Thank You to Jenny Levison for your awesome restaurant inspiration as well! Café Jonah + the Magical Attic was one of my faves. Rosetta's Kitchen in Asheville… the list goes on + on! (I am a menu-saver! ;))

More Gratitude: I also want to thank my amazing Kitchen Goddess Crew: Laura Grierson, Lotem Porat, Tatiana Graham, Kiana Prema, Julia Ahmadi, I love + appreciate you. Mia, thank you for your love + energy. Lamont, thank you for being our "Man!" Also, a special thanks to Celeste + Elysse, my first Kitchen Goddesses last year at the Chumash Village in Malibu! Shakti, Michelle, Rebecca, xoxoxo.

Special gratitude to Jillian Anderson, my cosmically-ordained writing partner for the past year! And to Gwyneth for facilitating the connection, and believing in books! To Dana Kramaroff for our writing buddy-ship + long-lasting sacred friendship! To Mom, for passing along a love of recipes, and for your amazing editing skills. For Grandma Bernice for looking this over, and giving me a loving kick. To Ariana, for having my back + all the connections made. To Naseem, Rosie, Atourina, Nichole, Sarah, Joey, and all the other support people along the way! Isis + Kailey, you are my doula + assistant doula at the end. What would we do without each other??!

Special thanks to Rose Park Roasters, my "office" + peaceful writing haven. Thank you for your smiles, for your positive vibes (and great music!) + of course, for the jasmine kombucha.

And thank you, Shiva Rea, for inspiring these particular menus, as I tuned into the energy of your beautiful retreats + the planet that we both envision. Thank you Karyn + all the others who helped make our experience beautiful in Malibu.

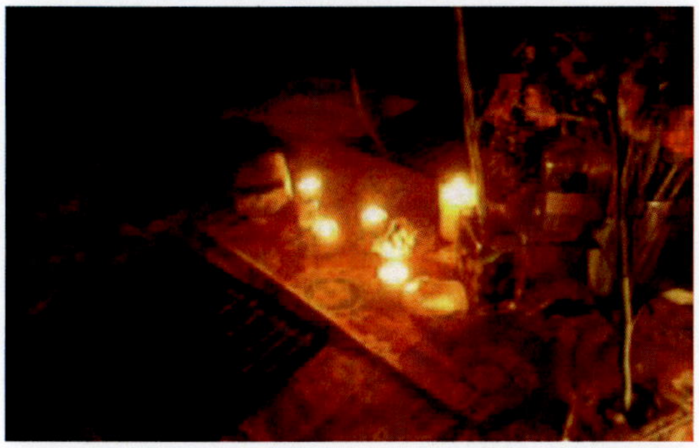

Tips of the Trade

Equipment + Different Knives/ Tools for Different Ingredients: My first love in the Kitchen, ever since I got one 11 years ago, is my Vitamix. A high-speed blender, a food processor with different blades. A food dehydrator, although you don't need one for any of these recipes. Some good knives, both flat-edge + serrated, fun stainless steel mixing bowls of various sizes, bamboo cutting boards. Some fun liquid + solid measuring cups + spoons. A great garlic press. Stainless steel pots + pans for cooking. Spatulas, rubber spatulas + bamboo spoons for mixing. These are all wonderful tools to have by your side.

Where to Source Ingredients/ Get Spices: A great place to buy spices is the bulk spice bin at your local co-op or health food store. This is always my first choice. Even sea salts can be purchased in bulk at the health food store. Frontier Herbs is a brand I love. When I was a working member of Sevananda Co-op in Atlanta, I worked in the Bulk Spice section. I would spend my 3 or 4 hours a week refilling spices, + it was fascinating, + I learned (+ smelled) so much! Try hanging out in the bulk Spice/ or Tea section of your favorite health food store. Guaranteed, you will learn something new! Try a spice you have never been exposed to yet! ;)

For a spice like Berbere, which is used in Ethiopian cooking, I went to my local Ethiopian restaurant to purchase this traditional spice blend from them! ;) The Berbere I used for the retreats came straight from a very magical local chef's mother in Ethiopia! How amazing! And the woman insisted on gifting it to me. Truly phenomenal, a magical blessing.

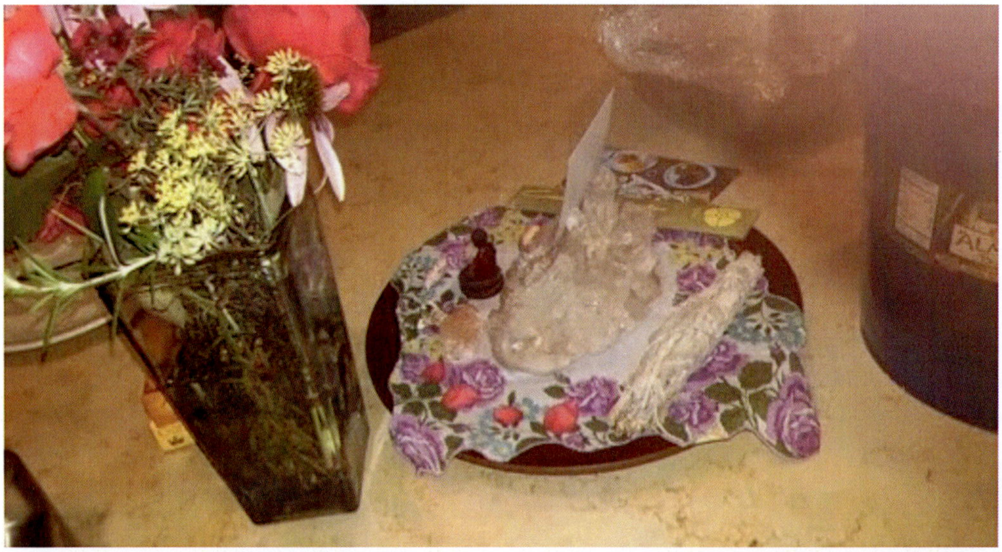

Math + Cooking: Little did I know that being a Math Nerd in elementary + middle school, winning the Math Award over + over again, embarrassingly, + having to go up on the stage in front of my classmates to accept it, would lead to a rewarding career in food + cooking! Math is essential for cooking for a big retreat. There is Recipe Conversion (taking a recipe that feeds 8, + making it feed 50) + then there is adding up all the produce for a giant order (1 T lemon juice + 2 tsp + 3 T = how many lemons??!). It is my joy using my Math Skillz for this loving Recipe Creation! ;) (There are always Calculators + Recipe Conversion Apps. ;))

Thoughts on Filtered Water: In an Ideal World, all of my water would come from a fresh, local spring. (See: findaspring.com) In real life, I often buy Reverse Osmosis or Alkaline Water, fill up giant 5 gallon jugs, + haul back to my home. If you're ready to invest, you can purchase a Reverse Osmosis or Alkaline Water system for your home. I was blessed in that the kitchen we used for Shiva Rea's yoga retreats was set up with a filtered water system. Hooray!

A Note about Soaking Beans: It's a wonderful idea to soak your beans. It makes them way more digestible, and also reduces cooking time. If you're lazy or low on time, you can buy canned organic beans, but I don't recommend it. I love to buy dry beans + soak them overnight before cooking them.

Here's how: 1) Soak dry beans in filtered water, covering them with twice as much water as beans, and leave on the countertop overnight. 2) In the morning, drain the soaking water + rinse beans 2 or 3 times, until they are foam-free + the water runs clear. 3) Now you are ready to cook your beans!

Soaking Grains + Rice: Same idea with Grains + Rice. Believe it or not, soaking your grains + rice reduces acids that can damage your teeth, + overall makes the grains more digestible. Spend time in a kitchen in India or other parts of the world, + people are soaking + fermenting everything, for better digestion. It's the natural, ancient way.

So, once again, here's how to do your overnight soaking: 1) Soak rice overnight in filtered water, covering the rice with twice as much water as rice. 2) In the morning, drain the soaking water, + give rice/ grains one rinse. 3) Now you are ready to cook your rice!

Soaking Nuts + Seeds: Nuts + seeds also require overnight soaking. I learned this as a Raw Food Chef. Soaking your nuts + seeds removes acids + enzyme inhibitors, + makes them more digestible. (Also, from a Chef's perspective, it changes their texture + makes them creamy + ready to blend into nut cheeses + patés.) Same thing goes for soaking nuts. I keep it simple + soak all nuts + seeds overnight. 1) Soak nuts/ seeds in filtered water, covering them with twice as much water as nuts/ seeds, and leave on the countertop overnight. 2) In the morning, drain the soaking water + rinse nuts/ seeds once, or until water runs clear. 3) Now your soaked nuts/ seeds are ready to use! If you don't use them right away, keep them in the fridge to stay fresh. They will last 5 (ish) days in the fridge.

Soaking Dried Fruit: Soaking dried fruit is a little different than beans, rice, + nuts, because you only need to cover dried fruit like raisins + sundried tomatoes, with enough water to barely cover the top. Otherwise, you will lose the flavor of your dried fruit. The fruit can be soaked overnight with filtered water, + unlike other soak-water which needs to be discarded, you can actually save the soak-water of dried fruit. Sundried tomato water is great for soups + salad dressings, + raisin or date water can be used for sweet drinks or desserts (just be careful of changing the texture ;)).

A Note About Sulfur-Free: It's important when purchasing your sundried tomatoes, organic raisins + dates, + other dried fruit, + even unsweetened shredded coconut, that they be Sulfur-Free. Sulfur dioxide is a preservative, + I choose to stay clear of preservatives when I cook. ;)

Sweeteners: My favorite all-time sweeteners right now (and yes, they change) are Raw Local Honey + Grade B Maple Syrup. I'm noticing lately that Grade B Maple Syrup has changed names, in some instances, to Grade A Dark Maple Syrup. I'm not sure why! ;) But keep an eye out for this!

Why do I love Raw Local Honey + Grade B Maple Syrup? Well, both of them are loaded with minerals + nutrients. Eating locally grown raw honey can be a great cure/ preventative measure for allergies, as the honey contains a homeopathic dose of local pollen. In the Master Cleanse, Grade B Maple Syrup is recommended, because it has the minerals + nutrients to keep you alive + nourished, when all you are consuming is lemon juice, cayenne, + filtered water. These sweeteners feel best to me! If you are strict Vegan + choose not to consume a bee product, feel free to sub with your favorite sweetener of choice! ;) I do my best to stay away from white sugar, unless I'm out + I just have to be part of the festivities! Honey + Maple Syrup are the sweeteners I actually buy, along with some Stevia extract.

About Salts: Regular table salt has actually been bleached + stripped of its nutrients. I know, that's hard to believe! But it's true. We live in a racist culture that wants to "whiten" everything, but actually, when your Himalayan Salt is pink or your Real Salt from Utah has brown speckles, this is a good thing! True, real sea salt is loaded with minerals that are replenishing to the body! Make sure to use Sea Salt, Pink Himalayan Salt, or Real Salt in place of standard Table Salt. I'm not crazy about iodized salt either, but that's just me! ;) TJ Maxx actually has quite a selection of Pink Himalayan Salt in their Housewares section; you should check it out sometime! ;)

Oils: Generally, I try to cook everything in Organic Coconut Oil. This is because coconut oil does not change its molecular structure when heated, whereas other oils do. Now, this is not to say I never cook with Olive Oil, because sometimes I love the flavor! But almost all of the recipes you see here use coconut oil to sauté the onions, etc. And olive oil is usually reserved for raw salads, or a topping after the fact. These are the only two oils I cook with. I love to use Toasted Sesame Oil as a flavoring to add into a dish right before serving. A restaurant I once worked at used Grapeseed Oil for frying, + this is a good choice too. Quality Oils = Quality YOU! ;)

Making Fresh-Squeezed Lemon Juice: I always recommend making your own fresh lemon (+ lime) juice. When I lived in Atlanta, I used to buy 16-oz bottles of freshly squeezed lemon or lime juice each week, for $3.99 a bottle! It was the best deal! Here, I've been juicing lemons + limes myself. An electric citrus juicer is great, or even one of those hand-held wooden citrus juicers to twist + squeeze out the nectar! I always, always use fresh, + never, ever lemon juice from a bottle on the shelf. Fresh ingredients = yummy food, + life-giving, healthy food!

"Chunks" aka. The Hippie Chef: In our Kitchen, Lotem + I quickly came up with a joke about me being a "Hippie Chef." (Love You Lotem! ;)) Whenever she would ask me how to cut the potatoes, or the tomatoes, or the avocados, I would say, "In Chunks!" Little chunks, big chunks, medium-size chunks…. I did not get formal training at a Chef's School! I learned through doing, + through working on ecovillages + farms. Chopping what we grew. Following recipe books. Taking classes + trainings here + there, working at restaurants + under people whose food + spirits I admired. (Thank You Jackie Graff! ;)) Therefore, mincing, chopping in ribbons, + julienning are terms I use here in the book, but I also lovingly include the Vocabulary of "Chunks!" Enjoy + laugh along with our Kitchen Goddess humor! We are hippies in the making! ;)

How to Chop Various Vegetables: Just a quickie about knives. I like to use a serrated edged knife for tomatoes, + a flat edged knife for just about everything else. See which knife is easiest for your chopping project, + go with that one! It's okay to try different sizes + types. ;) Always carry your knife face down + be loving!

Using Food Processor to Chop Garlic + Ginger: When making big batches, it can be helpful to use the food processor (with S blade) to chop your peeled garlic + ginger. Otherwise, ginger can be minced by hand with a knife + cutting board. And for garlic, I love to peel by hand + use a garlic press! Always fresh garlic, that I peel myself, for the ultimate fresh taste + vibration. Note: when using the food processor (or blender), always use a rubber spatula to spoon out the food, hands-free!

Timing + How to Prep Ingredients while Dishes are Cooking: One fun thing about cooking (rather than prepping raw foods) is that the foods cook themselves! You add ingredients, + sometimes there is an hour (or more) where a pot is just literally cooking on the stove. I like to multi-task, in this instance! Perhaps, while your rice is on the stove simmering, you can blend up a smoothie for tomorrow morning, or make a salad! While your onions are sautéing, you might be able to chop the next ingredient, such as kale or broccoli. See how you can maximize your time so you're not "sitting around waiting for a pot to boil." Plan your time + cooking can be quick + easy! I love listening to podcasts, music, + classes, while I cook!

Bowls I love to use: My favorite bowls are those stainless-steel mixing bowls. I've even been known to eat salads out of them, with chopsticks or my bare hands! I do have some plastic, but I prefer stainless steel or "natural" materials like glass, wood, or bamboo. See what you like, + go with it. Life is yours to design! You're in charge! ;)

Recipe Symbols:

Δ = Overnight Soaking
⊕ = Non-Vegan
♥= 80% or more, Raw
∇ = Sprouting

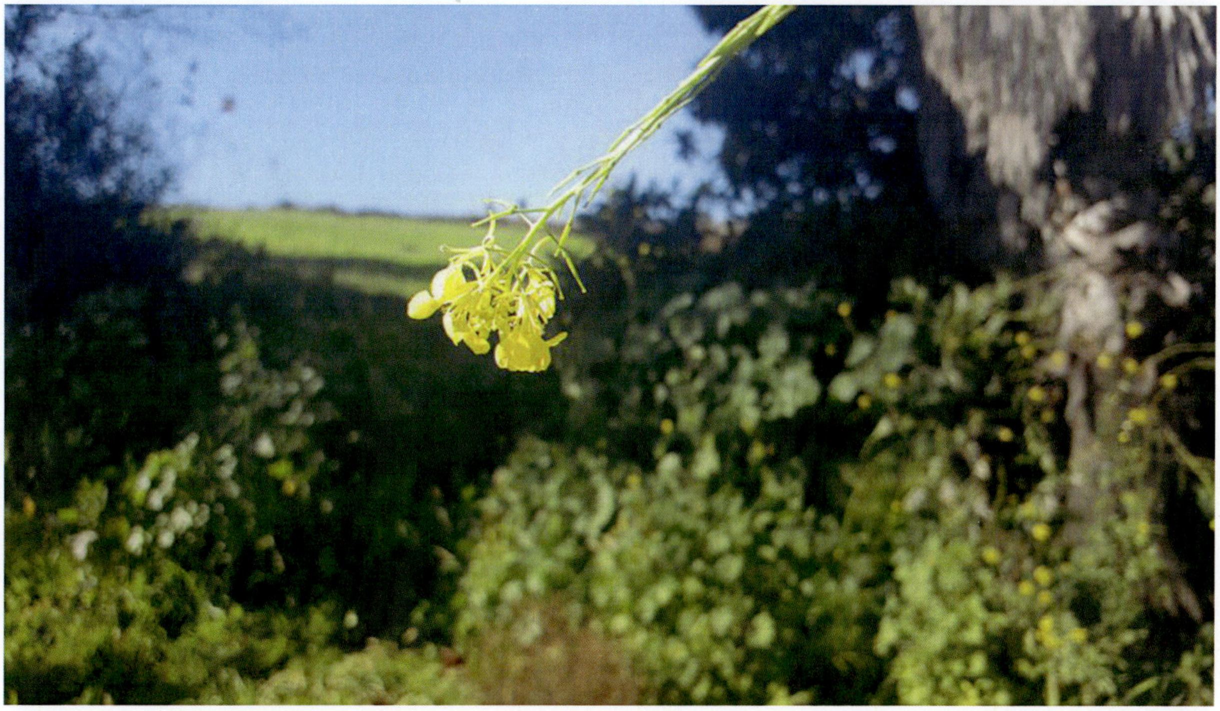

Ethiopian Feast

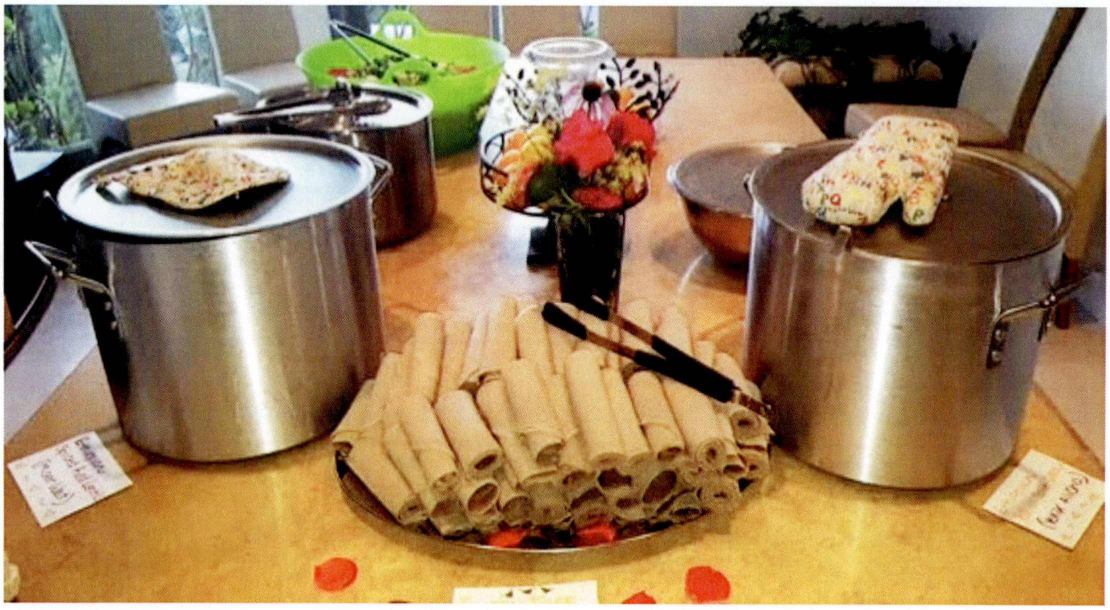

Note: I want to express my deep gratitude to Afya Ibomu, whose powerful vegan business in Atlanta has inspired me for years! Her vegan Ethiopian recipes from her gorgeous + delicious book, The Vegan Remix, have greatly inspired this particular meal!

ΔEthiopian Yellow Split Peas (Yekik Alicha) – inspired by Afya Ibomu's Yekik Alicha, The Vegan Remix
Serves 6
Time: 1 ½ hours

1 ½ c yellow split peas, dry
4 cups filtered water
1 T coconut oil
½ tsp turmeric powder
1 tsp sea salt
1 c onion, chopped into small "chunks"
3 cloves garlic, pressed or finely chopped
1 tsp fresh ginger, finely chopped
1/8 jalapeño, finely chopped

1) Soak split peas overnight w/ filtered water. Use twice as much water as split peas, as they will expand to soak up all the water!
2) The next day, drain water from split peas, + rinse 2-3 times with running water, to remove any residue + keep the beans fresh + easily digestible! Ideally the 3rd time, the water will run clear + they are ready to cook!
3) Cook yellow split peas in filtered water (again, twice as much water as split peas) along with a pinch of sea salt/ pink Himalayan salt.
4) Meanwhile in a separate pan, heat up coconut oil + sauté chopped onion, pressed garlic, finely chopped ginger, finely chopped jalapeño. Heat until the onion is clear.
5) When split peas come to a boil, add sautéed ingredients, along with turmeric powder, + continue to cook on low heat until split peas are soft (up to 1 hour).

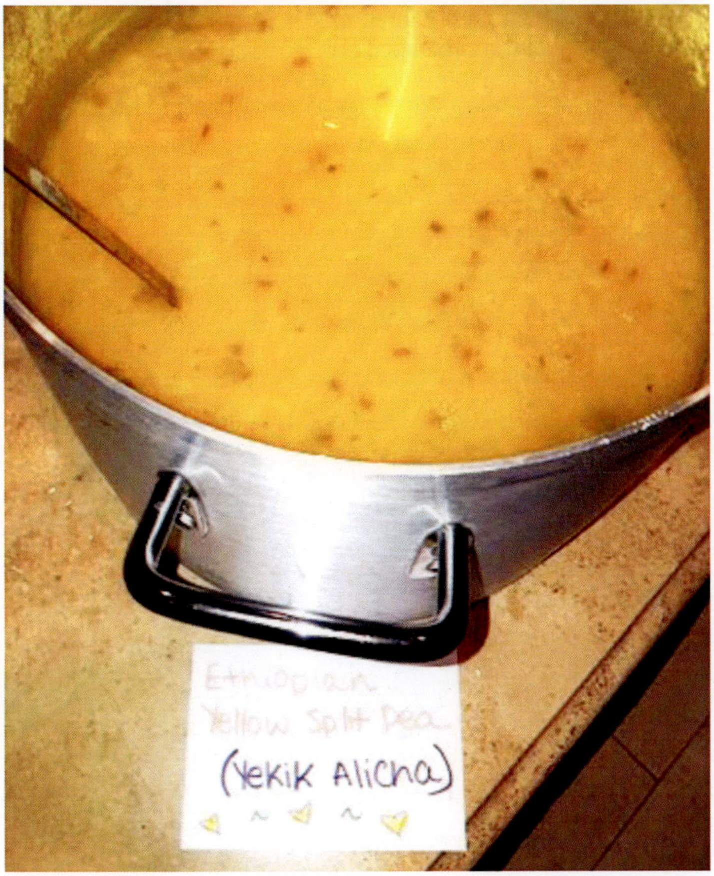

ΔEthiopian Spiced Red Lentils (Miser Wat) – inspired by Afya Ibomu's Miser Wat, The Vegan Remix
Serves 6
Time: 45 minutes - 1 hour

1 ½ c red lentils, dry
4 cups water
2 medium potatoes, chopped in 1 inch "chunks"
¼ c coconut oil
¼ c tomato, chopped in 1 inch "chunks"
1 c onion, chopped into small "chunks"
3 cloves garlic, pressed or finely chopped
1 tsp fresh ginger, finely chopped
1/8 jalapeño, finely chopped
1 T berbere blend, dry
2 tsp sea salt
1 tsp garam masala, dry
1 tsp paprika, dry
¼ tsp cayenne, dry

1) Soak red lentils overnight w/ filtered water. Use twice as much water as lentils, as they will expand to soak up all the water!
2) The next day, drain water from lentils, + rinse twice with running water, to remove any residue + keep the beans fresh + easily digestible! Ideally the 2nd time, the water will run clear + they are ready to cook!
3) Cook red lentils, along with potato "chunks" in filtered water (again, twice as much water as lentils) along with sea salt/ pink Himalayan salt.
4) Meanwhile in a separate pan, heat up coconut oil + sauté chopped onion, pressed garlic, finely chopped ginger, finely chopped jalapeño. Heat until the onion is clear.
5) When red lentils + potatoes come to a boil, add sautéed ingredients, along with berbere, garam masala, paprika, + cayenne. Continue to cook on low heat until everything is soft (30 more minutes).

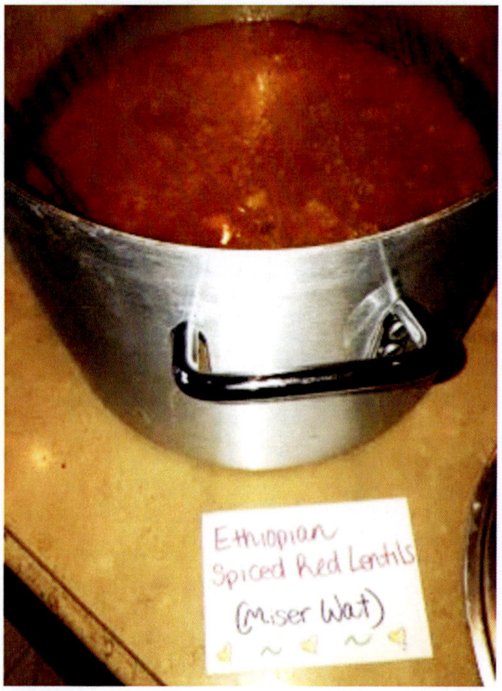

Ethiopian Carrot-Potato-Green Beans (Fasolia) – inspired by Afya Ibomu's Fosolia, The Vegan Remix
Serves: 5
Time: 30-40 minutes

¼ c coconut oil
1 c onion, chopped into small "chunks"
2 cloves garlic, pressed or chopped finely
1 T fresh ginger, chopped finely
1 c tomato, chopped into 1 inch "chunks"
3 medium potatoes, chopped into 1 inch "chunks"
3 large carrots, cut into rounds
1 lb fresh green beans, de-stemmed + cut in half
1 c filtered water
½ tsp coriander, dry
1 ½ tsp sea salt
¼ tsp black pepper
pinch berbere blend, dry

1) Put potato chunks, carrot rounds, green beans in a pot with filtered water + turn on High Heat.
2) Add tomato + sea salt (you can chop tomato while the first ingredients are cooking ;))
3) Meanwhile in a separate pan, heat up coconut oil + sauté chopped onion, pressed garlic, finely chopped ginger. Heat until the onion is clear.
4) When water in pot begins to boil, turn down to low heat. Add sautéed ingredients, along with all dry spices.
5) Continue to cook until vegetables are soft!

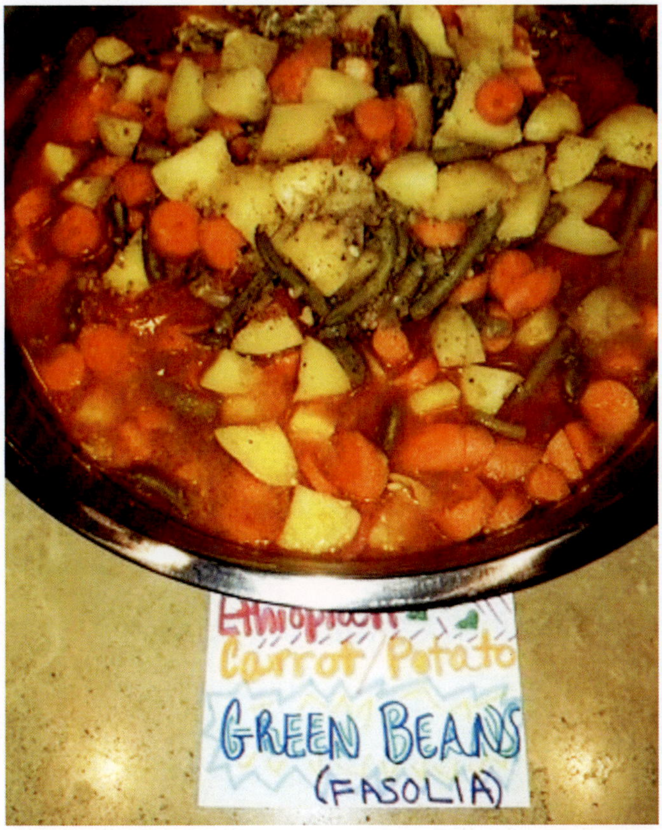

Ethiopian Cooked Greens (Gomen) – inspired by Afya Ibomu's Gomen, The Vegan Remix
Serves: 4
Time: 20 minutes

1 lb collard greens, fresh, julienned into ribbons (de-stem or leave the stem on, up to you! ;))
1/3 c coconut oil
1 c water
1 c onion
4 cloves garlic, pressed or chopped finely
1 T fresh ginger, chopped finely
1 c tomato, cut into 1 inch "chunks"
1 c bell pepper, minced
1 tsp sea salt
1 tsp ground cardamom, dry
½ tsp ground cumin
¼ tsp ground allspice
¼ jalapeño, fresh

1) In the bottom of a pot large enough to hold collards, heat up coconut oil + sauté chopped onion, pressed garlic, finely chopped ginger, + jalapeño. Heat until the onion is clear.
2) Next, add minced red bell pepper + tomato chunks.
3) Add half the collard greens, along with salt, + cook down. Add cumin, cardamom, + allspice.
4) As collards cook down + there is more room in the pot, add 2nd half + cook everything down.
5) Stir + eat!

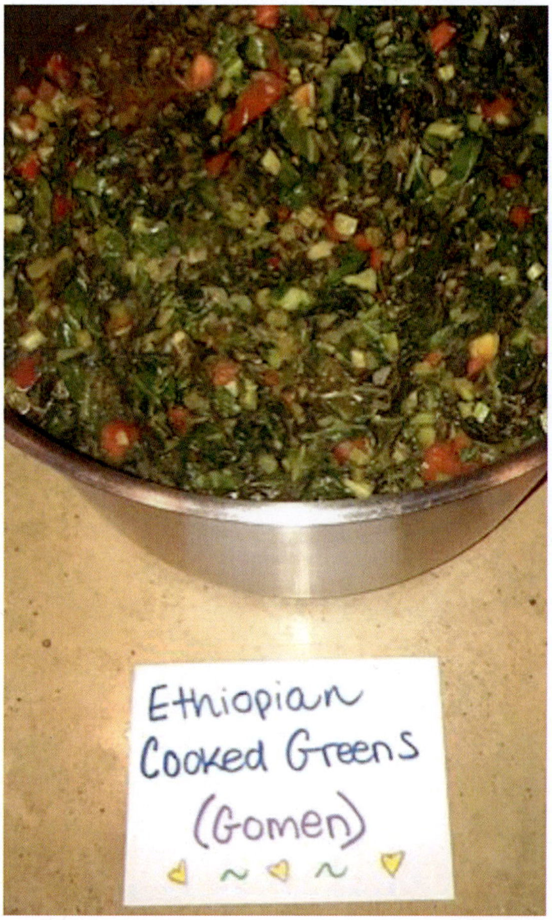

♥Butter Lettuce + Tomato Salad (Ethiopian Style)
Serves: 4
Time: 15 minutes

1 head butter lettuce, washed + broken into bite-size pieces
1 tomato, cut into 2-inch "chunks"
1/3 lemon, squeezed into juice
1 T olive oil
¼ tsp sea salt

1) Toss everything together!
2) Serve on top of injera, along with everything else!

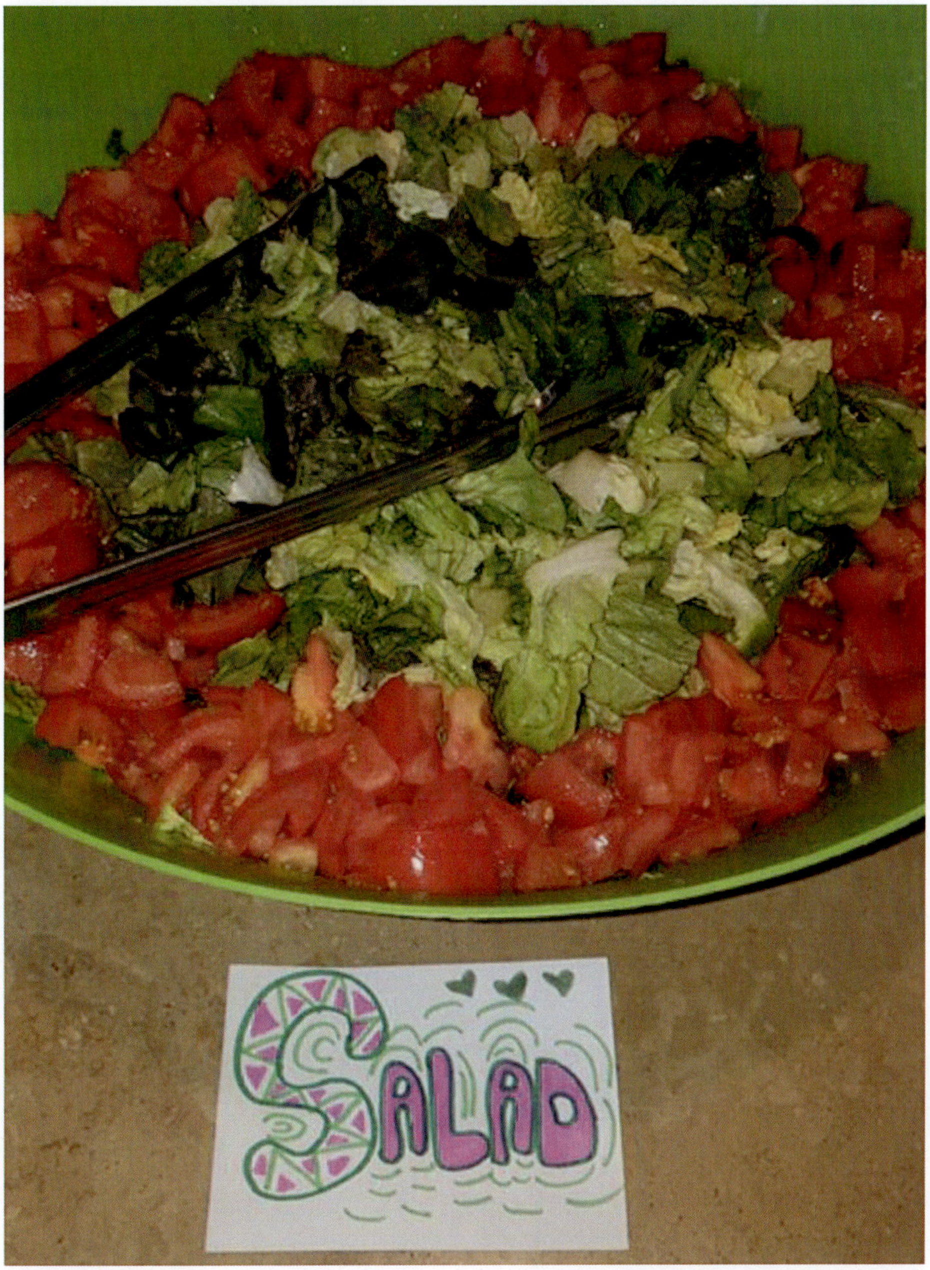

Where to get Gluten-Free Injera + How Much Per Person:

I recommend ½ full injera per person (Usually a full round injera is rolled + then cut into 2-3 pieces each). So, 1-2 rolls per person. (I know this doesn't sound like a lot, but we've had a lot of wasted injera giving each person a full round, + even after making "Injeramisu" our version of Bread Pudding/ Tiramisu, we still had to throw some injera away. ½ per person is the perfect amount for a big event. At home, or for a small dinner party, you can try a full injera per person + serve everything on the round injera, just like you would experience at an Ethiopian restaurant.)

The last Injera I bought was from an amazing all-Vegan Ethiopian restaurant near UCLA/ Downtown LA, called Azla. Their injera is 100% gluten-free! (Not all is.) I learned, sadly, that teff flour, a naturally gluten-free flour that injera is made out of, isn't the same here in the U.S. as it is in Ethiopia + doesn't bind as well. Therefore, many Ethiopian restaurants add a pinch of wheat or barley flour to their injera, to give it a better consistency. Azla uses quinoa flour to add to their teff. ;)

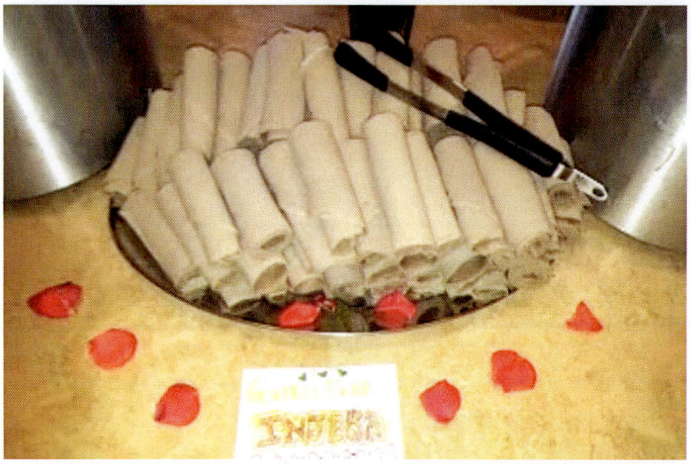

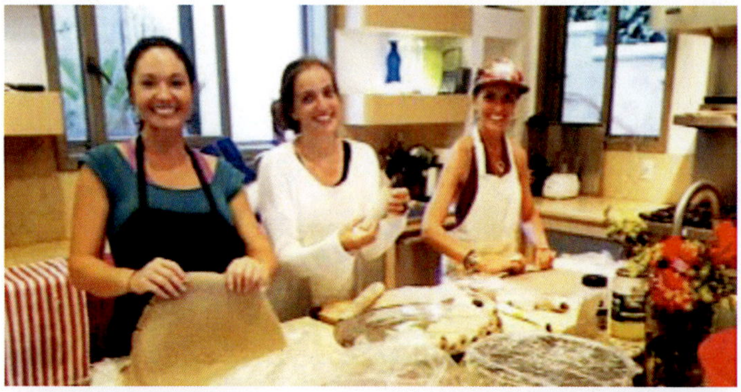

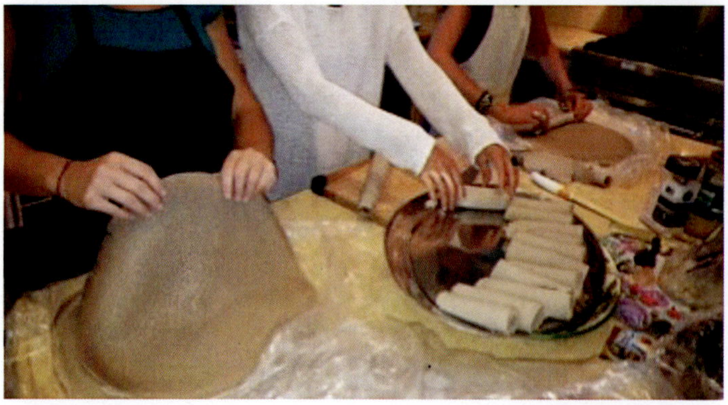

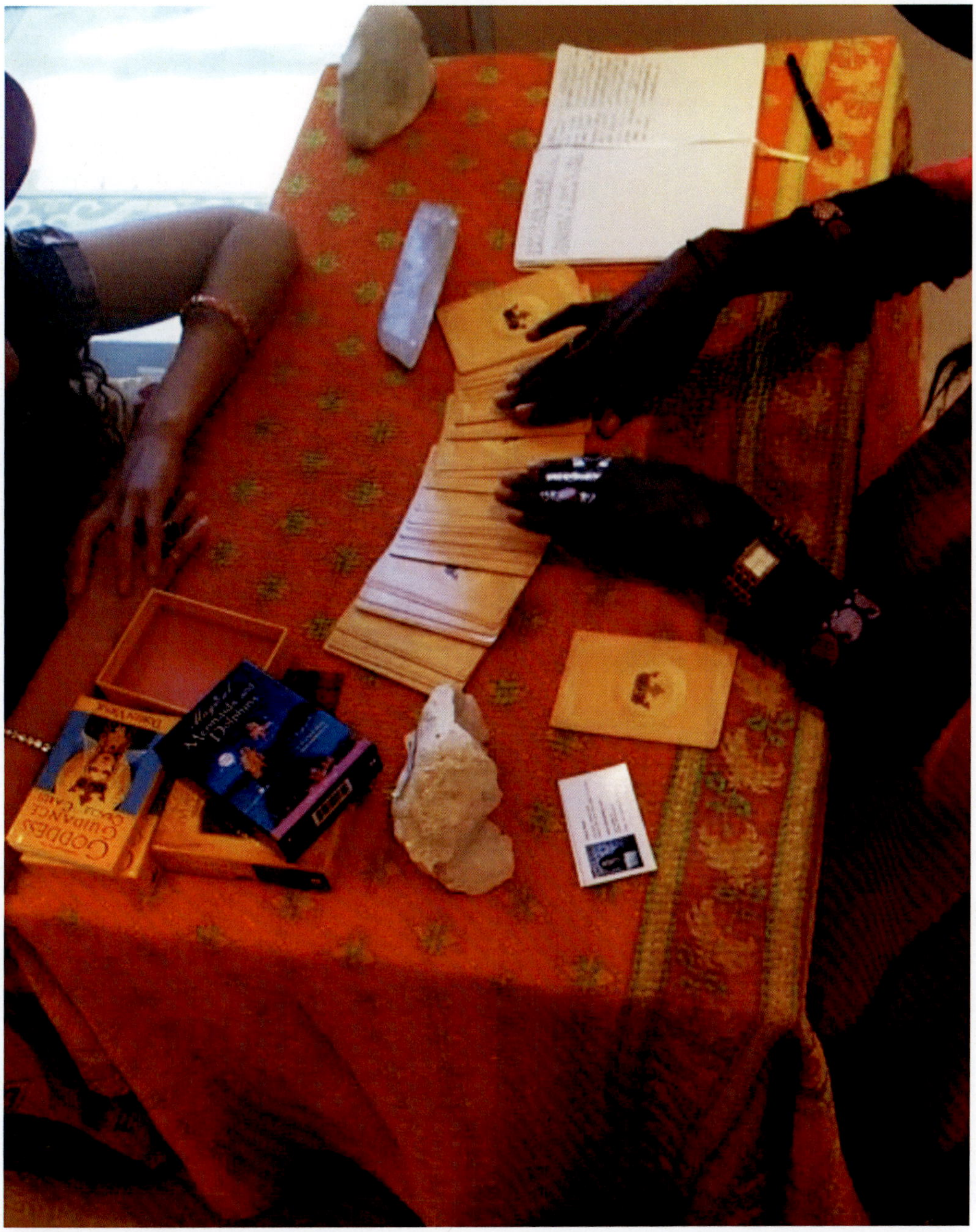

Island Tribe gorgeous hand model ♥

Mediterranean Lunch

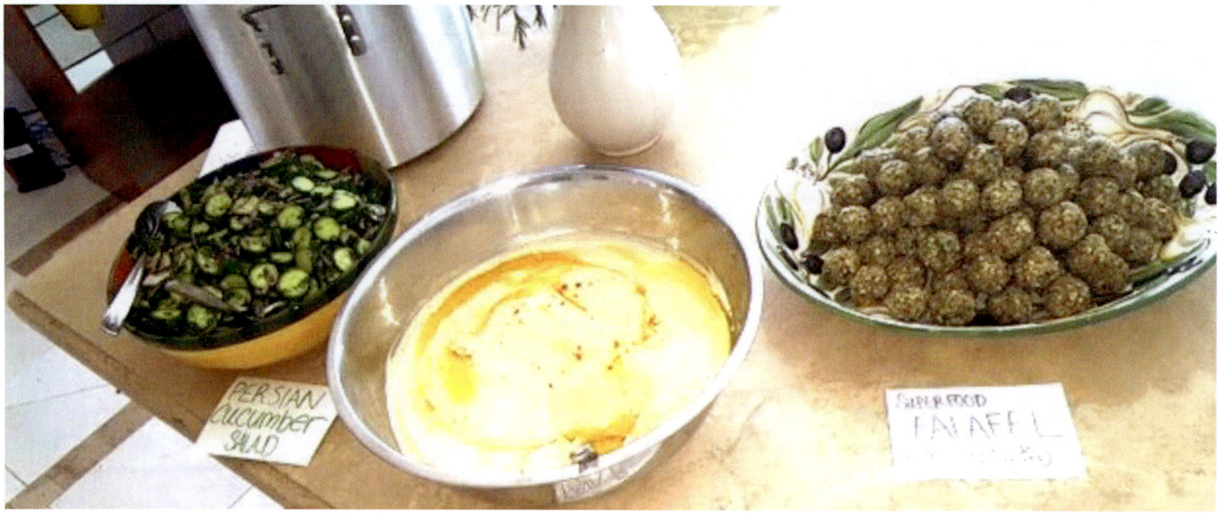

Quinoa Tabouli
Serves: 6
Time: 1 hour (will need to cook quinoa the day before)

4 c quinoa, cooked (start with 1 1/3 cups dry quinoa, cook with 2 2/3 cup filtered water)
1 bunch parsley, chopped finely
1 cucumber, chopped in small "chunks" (optional)
1 medium tomato, chopped in small "chunks"
1 tsp sea salt
2 T olive oil
3 T fresh-squeezed lemon juice
3 T fresh mint, chopped finely
2 cloves garlic, pressed or chopped finely

1) Cook quinoa the night before, then chill.
2) Add all other ingredients, stir + eat!

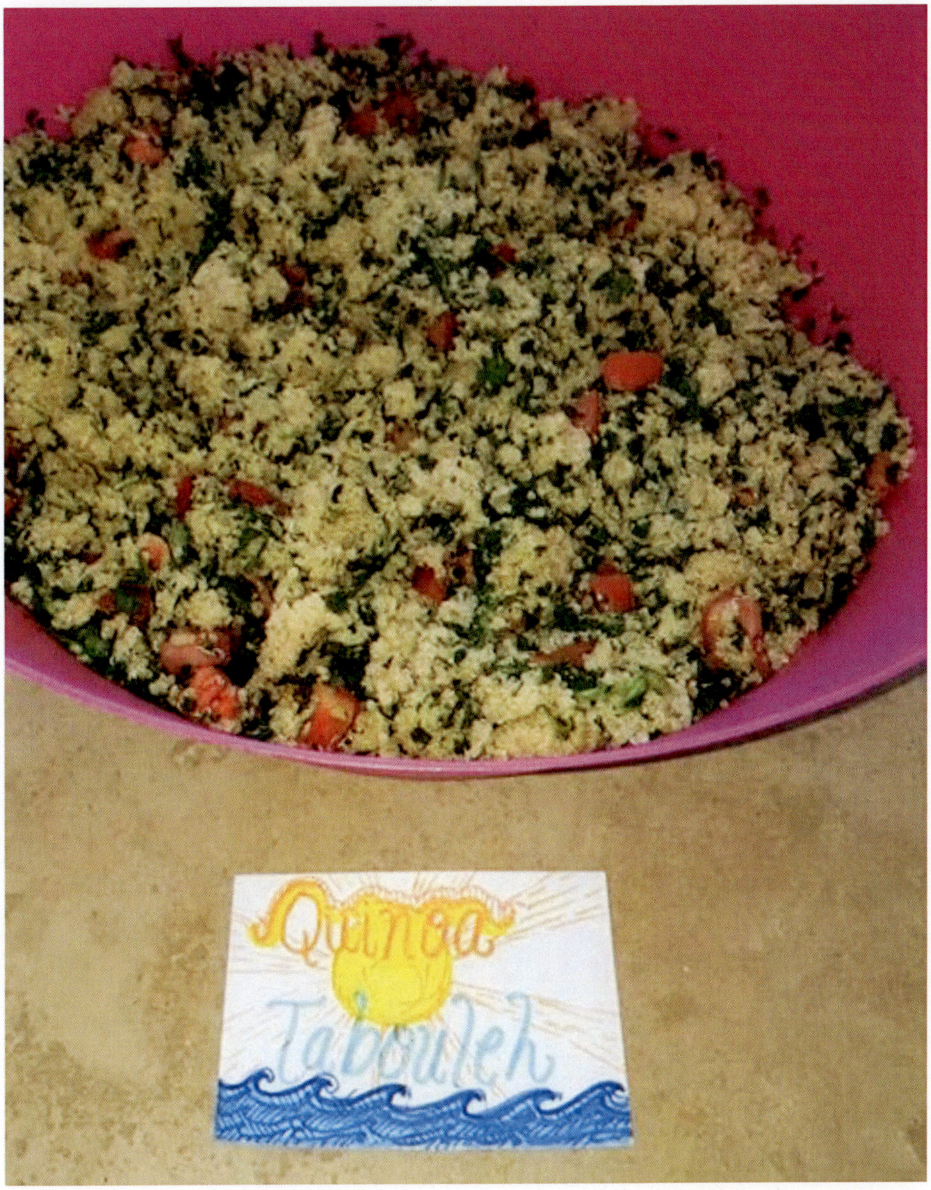

♥Cucumber Salad

Serves: 6
Time: 15 minutes

3 large cucumbers, chopped into medium “chunks” or thinly sliced rounds
1 T olive oil
1 T fresh-squeezed lemon juice
3 sprigs fresh mint, chopped finely
1/2 tsp sea salt
½ small red onion, sliced thinly
2 sprigs fresh dill, chopped finely

1) Slice cucumbers thinly into rounds.
2) Thinly slice red onions.
3) Chop fresh herbs in food processor.
4) Mix everything else together + enjoy!!

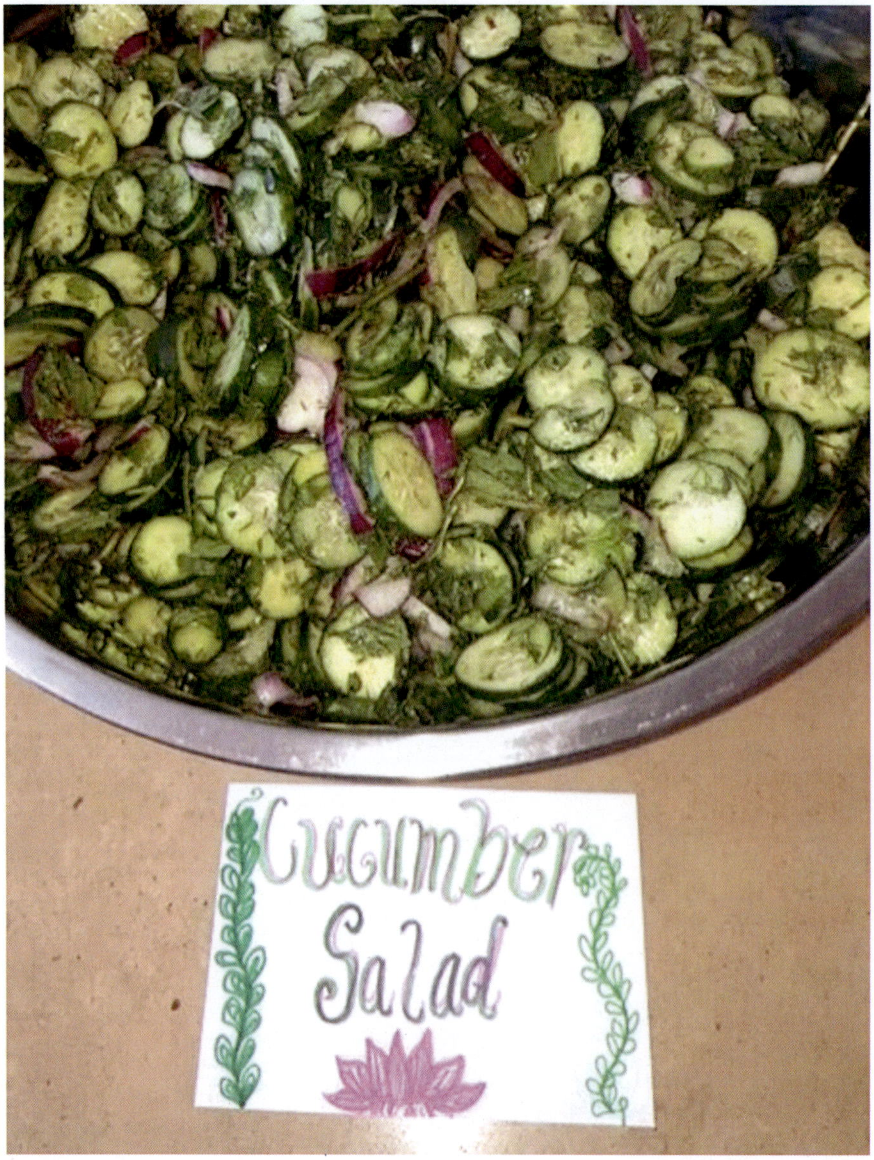

ΔFava Bean Hummus
Serves: 6
Time: 1 hour to cook beans, 15 minutes to make recipe (will need to start soaking beans 2 days before)

2 ½ c fava beans, cooked (1 cup dry)
1 c tahini (I love Maranatha, Once Again, Rejuvenative Foods, or Artisana brands) – can be raw or toasted
2 cloves garlic, pressed/ minced
¼ cup fresh-squeezed lemon juice
1 T sea salt
2 T olive oil
1 tsp cumin powder
¼ tsp ground black pepper
¼ c water

1) Soak 1 c dry fava beans overnight in 2 cups filtered water.
2) The next morning, drain + rinse beans a few times. Then cook drained beans in 2 cups filtered water, with a pinch of sea salt. Chill beans when done.
3) The next day, in Food Processor: Process garlic first, then beans. Then add tahini + all other ingredients + process till smooth. Yum Yum!!! ☺

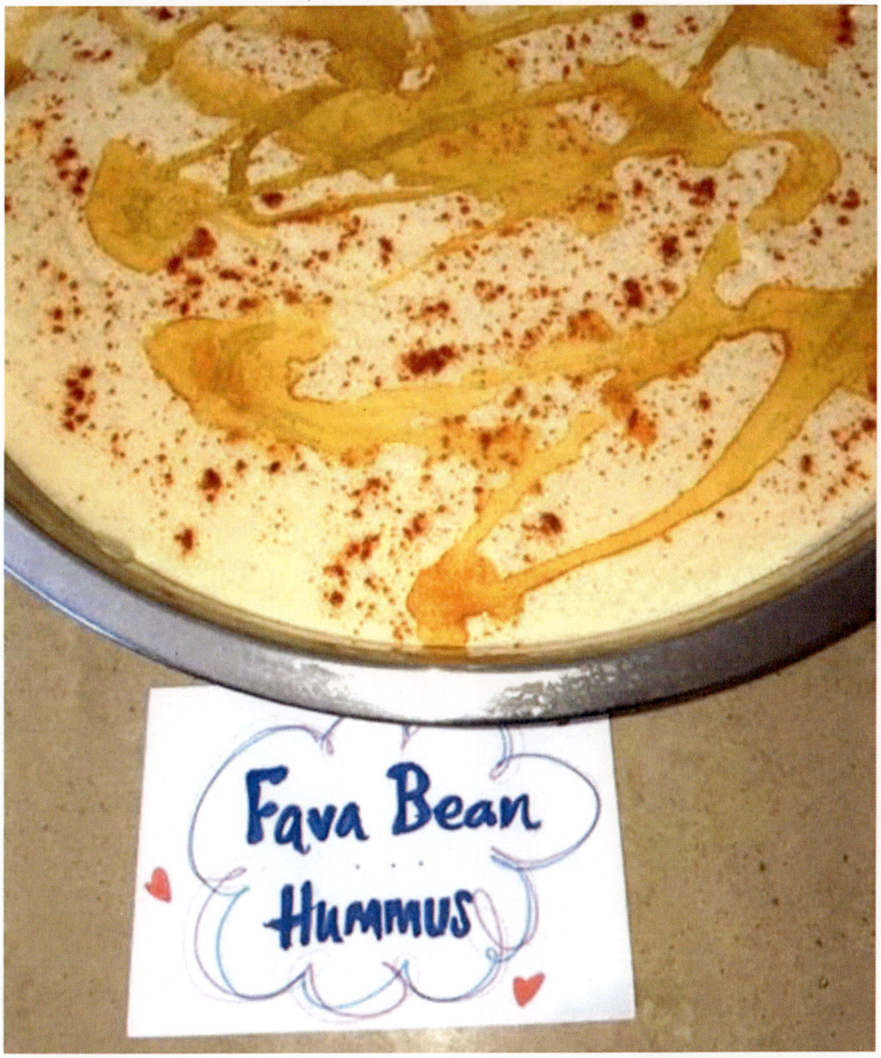

♥ΔRaw Falafel

Serves: 10
Time: 30 minutes (will need to soak nuts the night before)

2 c soaked walnuts
2 c soaked almonds
1 c Raw tahini
½ c parsley, finely chopped
2 T olive oil
3 cloves garlic
2 T dried oregano
1 T sage powder
1 tsp ground black pepper
1 T sea salt

1) Soak almonds + walnuts overnight. The next morning, drain + rinse nuts.
2) Food process garlic first, then almonds + walnuts. (Tip: Fill processor up only halfway for grace + ease in processing.) Pour ingredients into bowl.
3) Add tahini + all other ingredients into bowl. Then mash together with Reiki loving hands till all is blended together evenly + smooth. (You may use plastic gloves if making commercially.)
4) Roll into falafel-size balls + eat! (no dehydrating needed! ;))

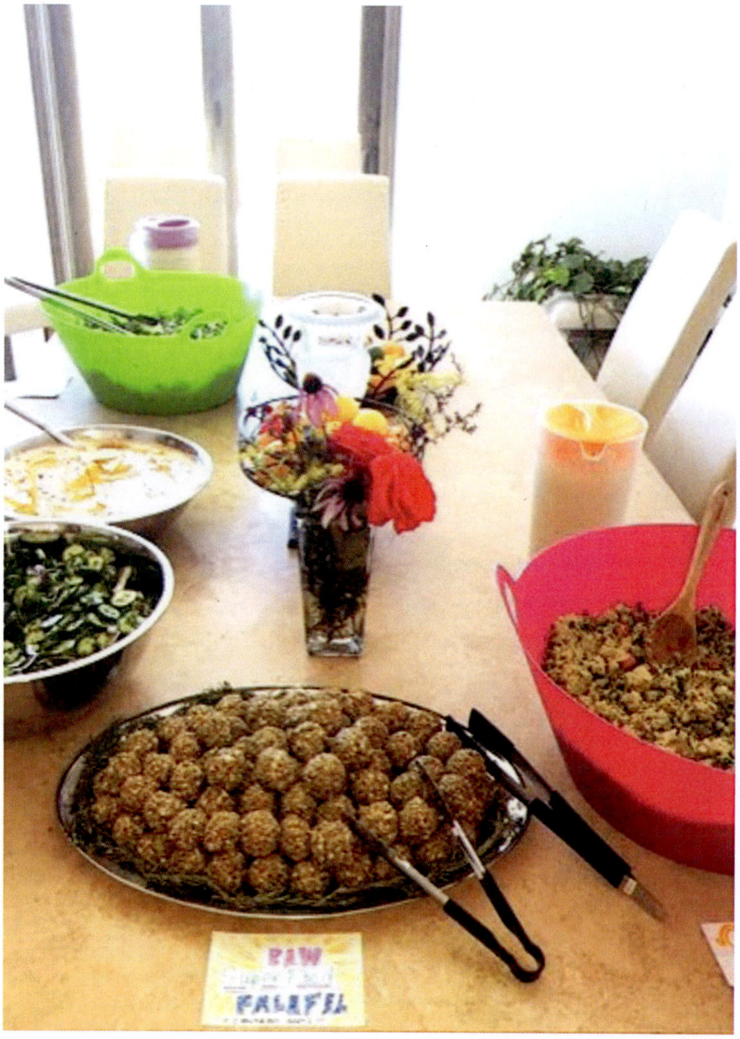

♥Tahini Dressing (The Ultimate!)

Serves: 10
Time: 15 minutes

1 jar Tahini (I love Maranatha, Once Again, Rejuvenative Foods, or Artisana brands) – can be raw or toasted
1 c fresh-squeezed Lemon juice
2 T sea salt
1/3 bunch fresh dill
1/8 t cayenne powder
½ c olive oil
4 cloves garlic
filtered water

1) Put all ingredients in blender (Vitamix) except for water.
2) Then add water + fill Vitamix to 8-cup line.
3) Blend + enjoy!

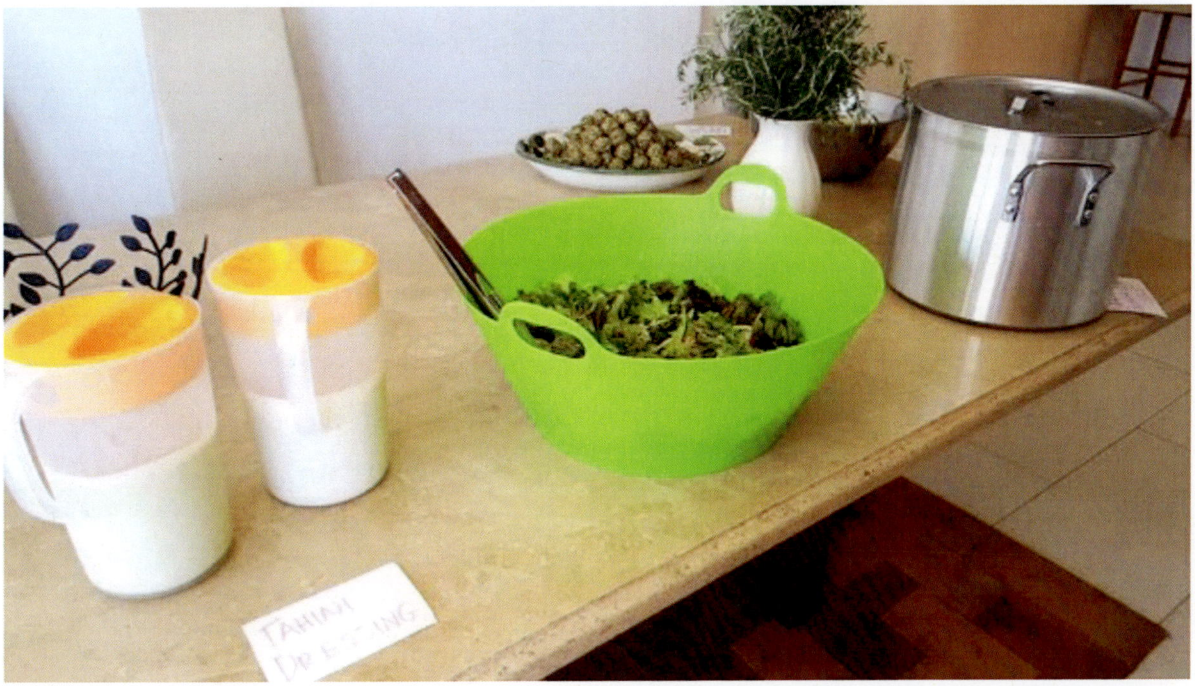

♥Halvah
Serves: 8
Time: 15 minutes (to make recipe), 1 hour (to chill before serving)

1 cup Honey (I love Raw Local honey – the best!)
½ cup Tahini (I love Maranatha, Once Again, Rejuvenative Foods, or Artisana brands) – can be raw or toasted
¼ cup slivered Almonds

1) Food process honey + tahini until creamy + well-mixed.
2) Pour into a glass baking dish + top with slivered almonds.
3) Chill in fridge/ freezer to "set" for 1 hour. Then cut into small squares + serve!

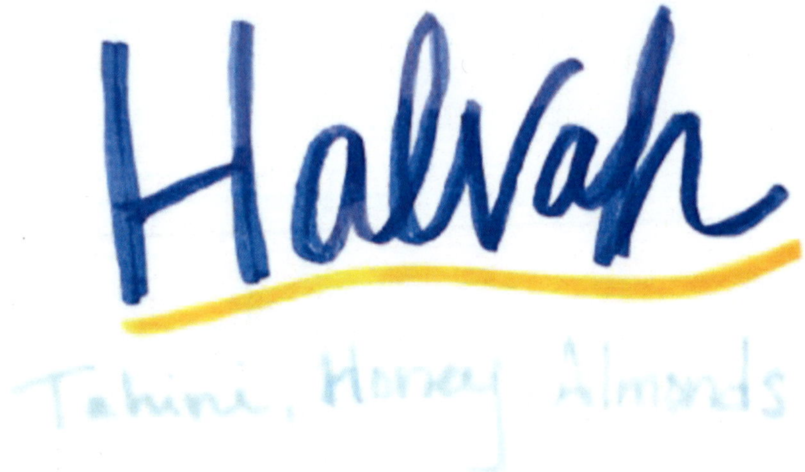

Caribbean Soul

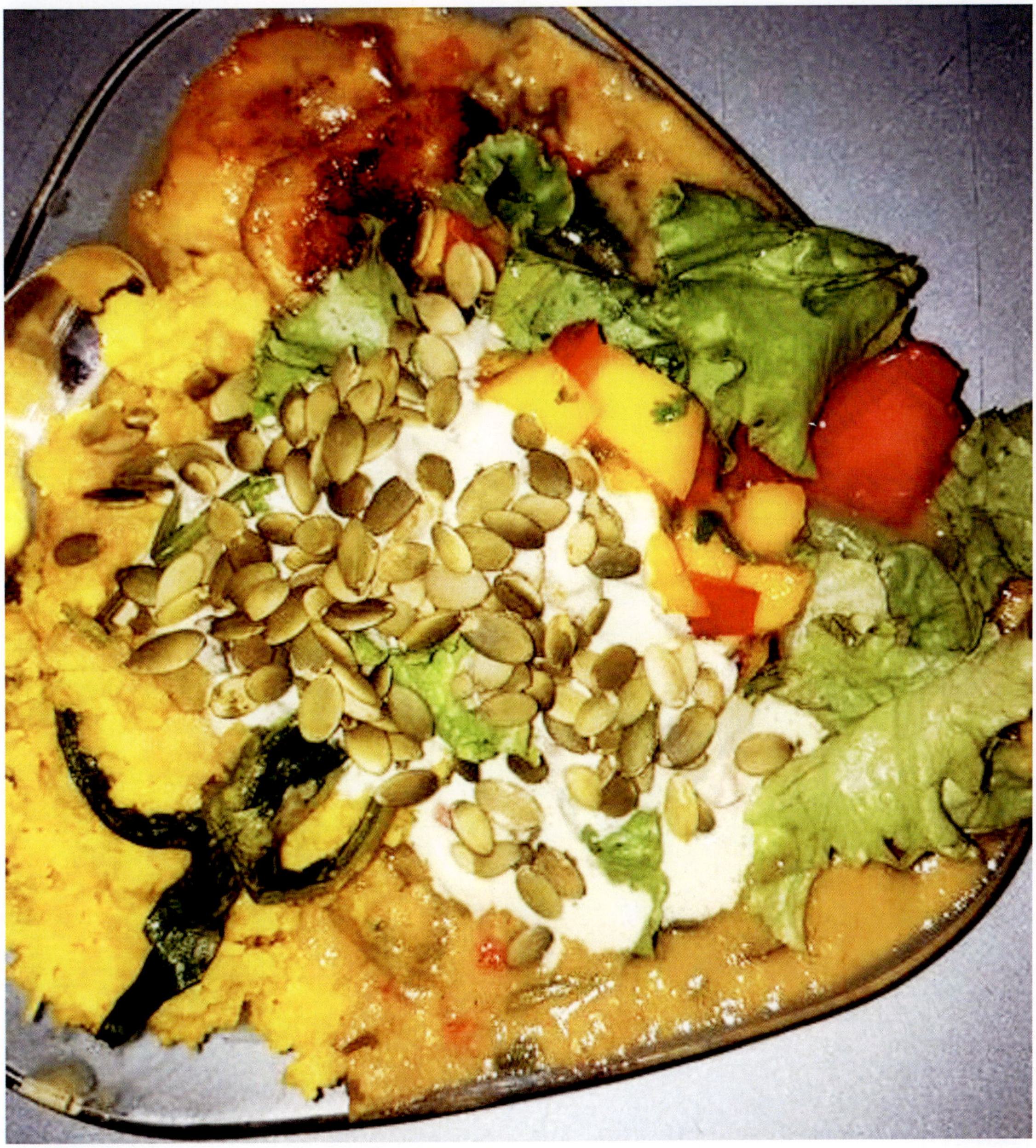

∆Yellow Coconut Rice
Serves: 4
Time: 1 hour (rice will need to be soaked the night before)

1 ½ c brown rice, cooked (1/2 cup dry)
1 can coconut milk (best price to get Organic Canned Coconut Milk is Trader Joe's!)
1 ½ c filtered water
1 tsp turmeric powder
1 tsp sea salt
2 ½ T shredded coconut, unsulfured (Trader Joe's makes a great organic bagged shredded coconut)

1) Soak rice overnight.
2) Cook soaked rice w/ 1 part rice, 1 part water. (Rice will have plumped up, where normally ratio would be 2-3 parts water to 1 part rice.)
3) When rice is cooked, add turmeric, sea salt, coconut milk, shredded coconut.
4) Stir until well mixed + turmeric is evenly distributed. Mmm!!!!

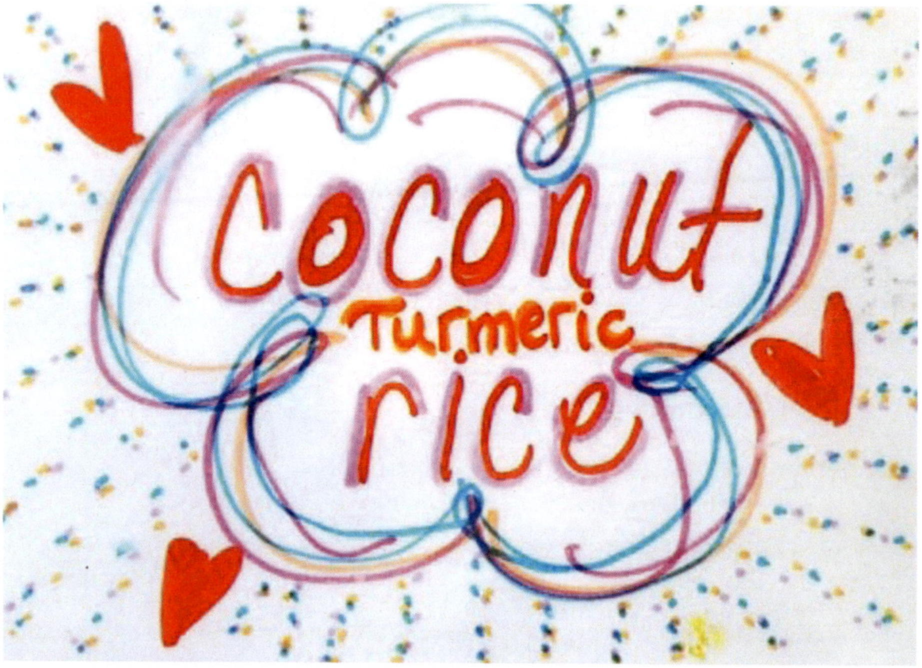

Fried Plantains
Serves: 4
Time: 15 minutes

2 plantains, ripe
1 T coconut oil
pinch sea salt

1) Cut ripe plantains in wide chunks at an angle.
2) Fry in coconut oil over medium-high heat. Flip to cook both sides to brown.
3) Sprinkle both sides with sea salt.
4) Enjoy the decadence!!

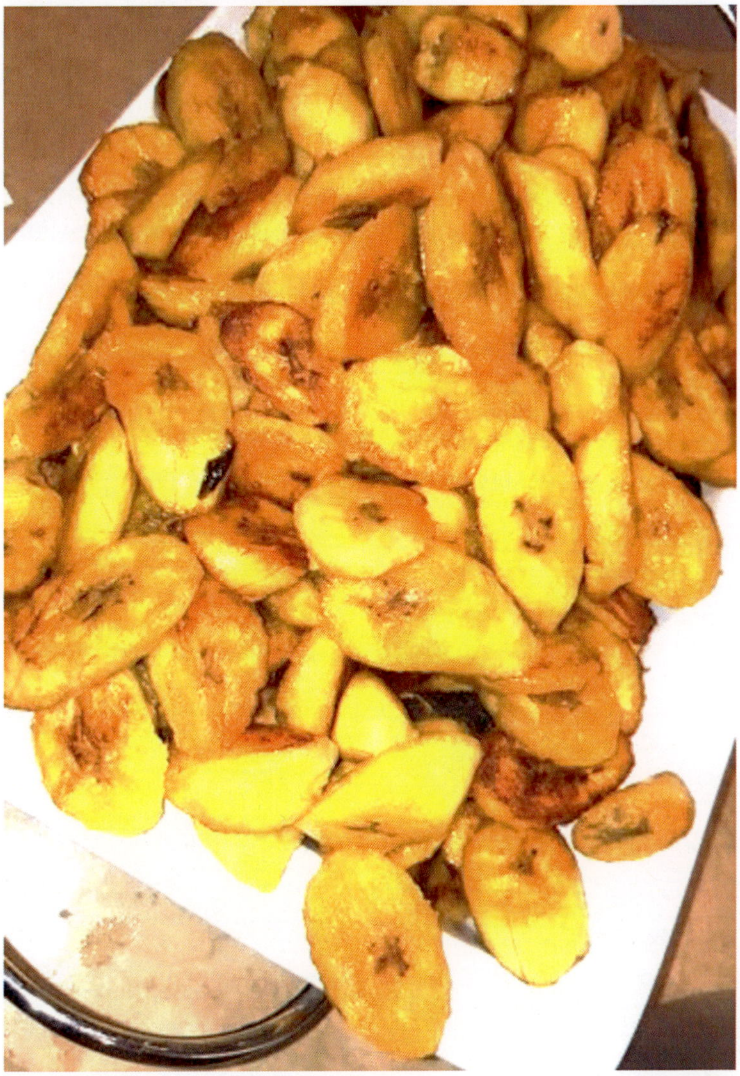

ΔCurry Red Lentils (Caribbean)

Serves: 6
Time: 1 hour

1 T coconut oil
1 large yellow onion, diced
2 cloves garlic, pressed/ minced
1 T ginger, finely chopped
1 T curry powder
½ tsp red pepper flakes
4 cups filtered water
1 can coconut milk
2 cups tomatoes, chopped into chunks
1 ½ c dry red lentils
1 bunch fresh spinach, washed + chopped into ribbons
pinch sea salt
pinch ground black pepper
1/3 bunch fresh cilantro, finely chopped

1) Soak red lentils overnight w/ filtered water. Use twice as much water as lentils, as they will expand to soak up all the water!
2) The next day, drain water from lentils, + rinse twice with running water, to remove any residue + keep the beans fresh + easily digestible! Ideally the 2nd time, the water will run clear + they are ready to cook!
3) Cook red lentils in filtered water (again, twice as much water as lentils) along with sea salt/ pink Himalayan salt.
4) Meanwhile in a separate pan, heat up coconut oil + sauté chopped onion, pressed garlic, finely chopped ginger. Heat until the onion is clear.
5) When red lentils come to a boil, add sautéed ingredients, along with chopped tomatoes, spinach, coconut milk, curry powder, red + black pepper. Continue to cook on low heat until everything is soft (30 more minutes). Just before serving, stir in chopped cilantro.

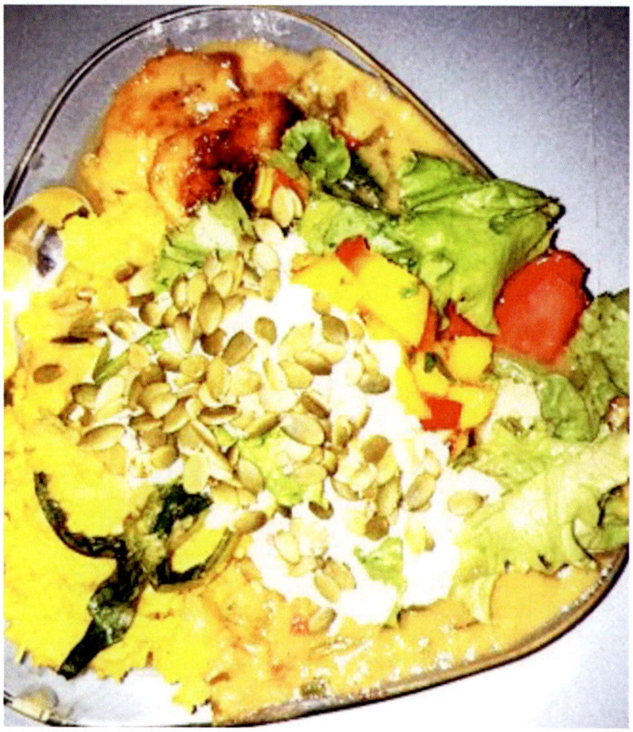

♥Green Salad
Serves: 4
Time: 15 minutes

1 head green/ red leaf lettuce, washed + broken into bite-size pieces
½ cucumber, thinly sliced into rounds
½ container Sunflower Sprouts

1) Arrange lettuce in a circular salad bowl.
2) Decorate with cucumber slices + sunflower sprouts in a mandala around the edges of the bowl.
3) Enjoy with Cashew Ranch dressing! Simple + Easy!

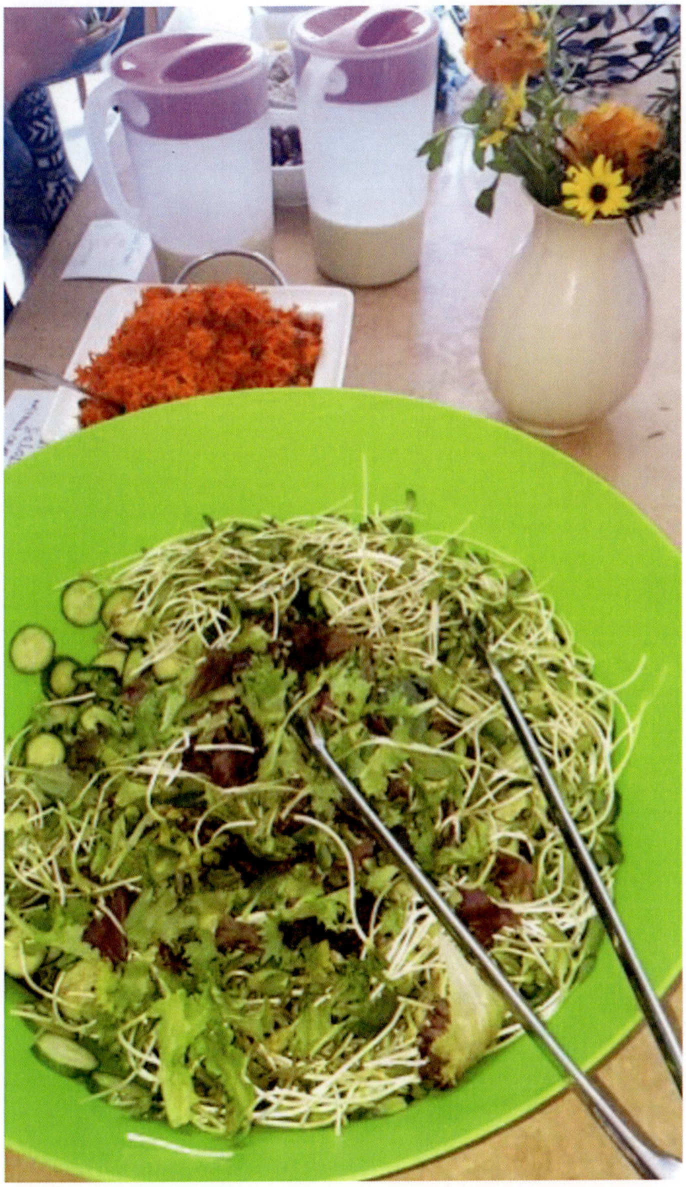

♥ΔCashew Ranch Dressing

Serves: 15 (great to save for 2-3 days!)
Time: 15 minutes

2 c Cashews, soaked
½ bunch fresh dill OR 2 T dried dill
1/4 c fresh-squeezed lemon juice
1 t sea salt
filtered water

1) Soak cashews overnight. Then drain + rinse cashews.
2) Put all ingredients except filtered water into the blender (Vitamix).
3) Add water up to the 4-cup line.
4) Blend + Enjoy!

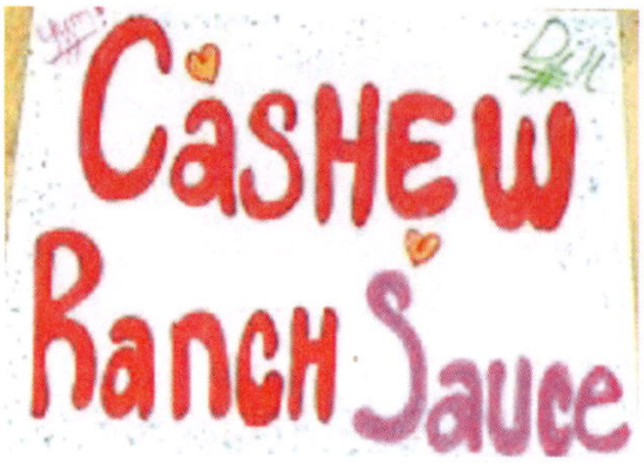

♥Mango Salsa
Serves: 6
Time: 30 minutes

3 mangoes, peeled + chopped into "chunks"
¾ c red bell pepper/ or tomato, finely chopped
½ c red onion, finely chopped
1 clove garlic, pressed/ minced
¼ jalapeño pepper, finely minced
2 T fresh-squeezed lime juice
½ tsp sea salt
¼ tsp ground black pepper
3 T fresh cilantro, finely chopped
1 T olive oil (optional)

1) Cut mango into small-medium "chunks."
2) Chop bell pepper, onion, cilantro, jalapeño.
3) Add all other ingredients + stir! Yum!

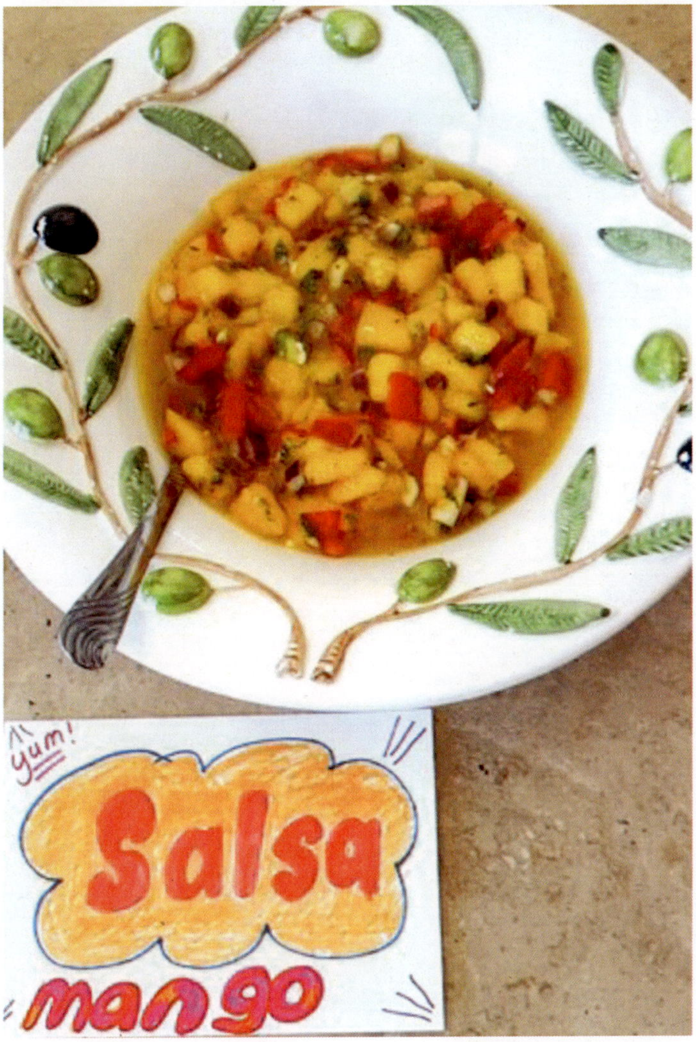

Salad Bar Extravaganza

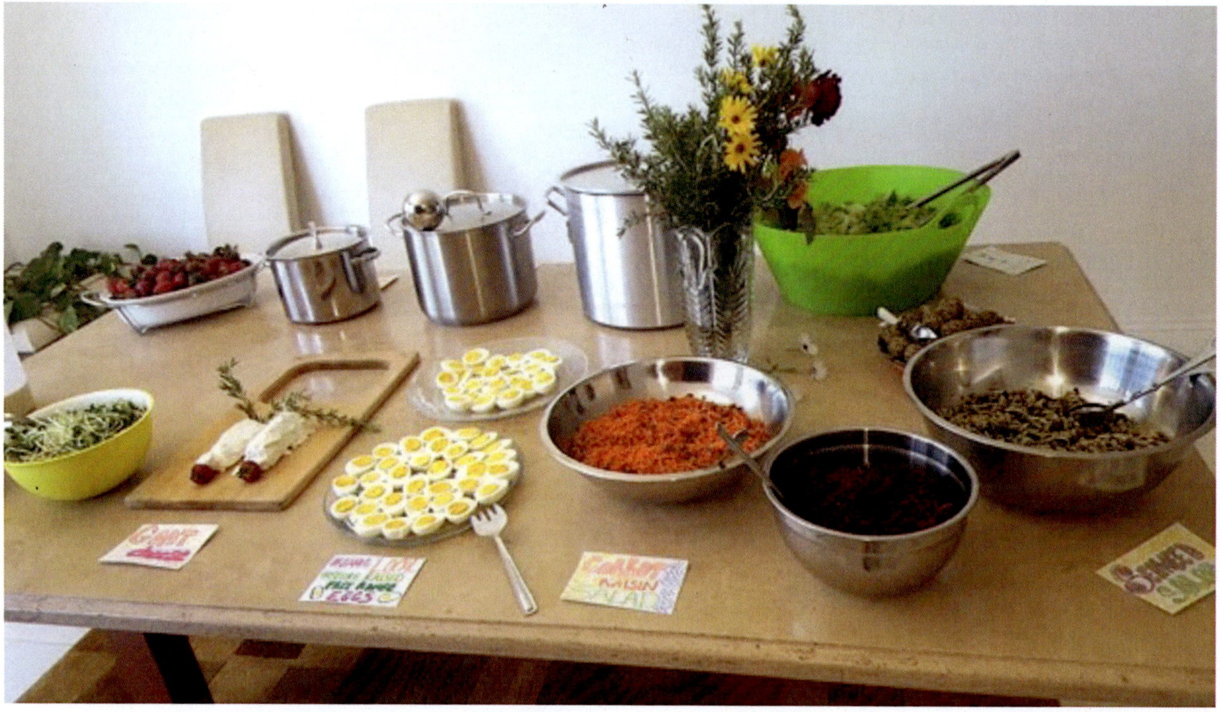

♥Green Salad for Salad Bar

Serves: 8
Time: 15 minutes

2 heads Leafy Green Lettuce, washed + torn/ chopped into bite-size pieces
2 avocado, sliced
3 tomatoes, cut into "chunks"
2 cups sunflower sprouts
2 cucumbers, thinly sliced into rounds or cut into bite-size "chunks"

1) Wash lettuce + break into bite-size bits, place into salad bowl.
2) Decorate top of bowl in "mandala" rows, a row of avocado, tomato, sunflower sprouts, + cucumber! It can be concentric circles with avocado in the middle, sprouts on the outside, etc.

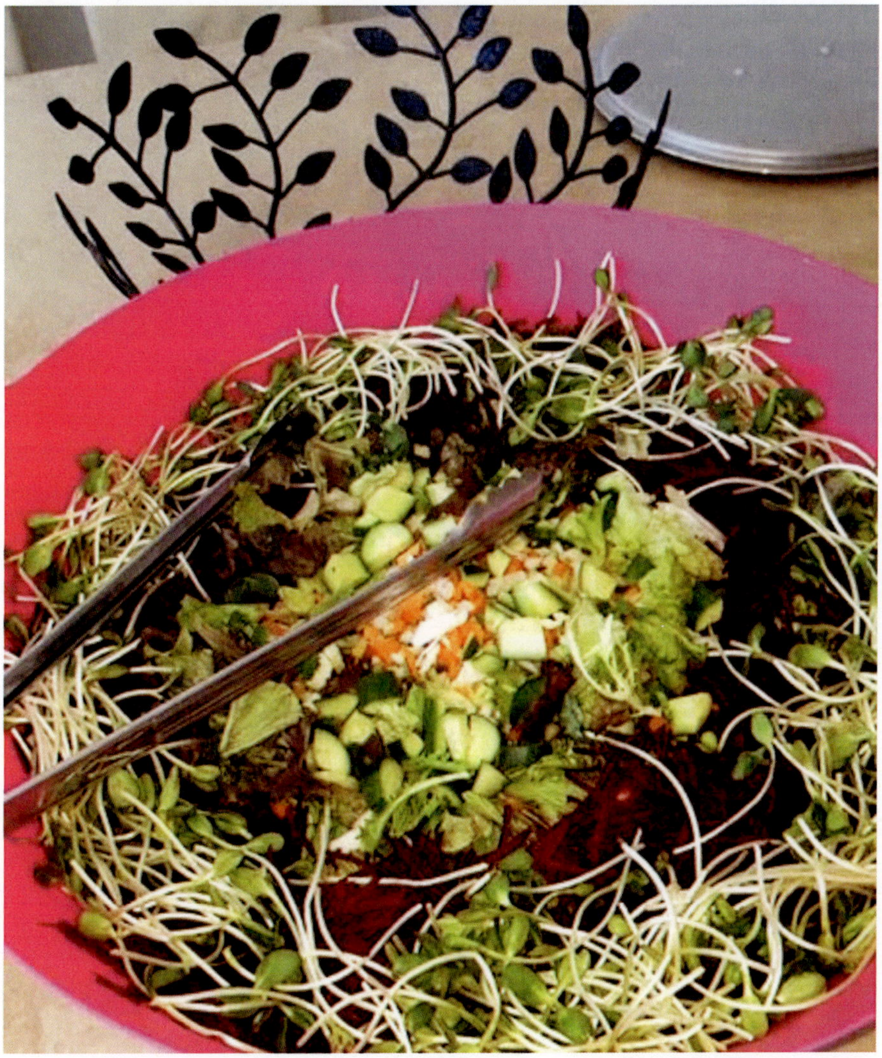

♥ΔAlmond Tuna

Serves: 8
Time: 20 minutes (overnight soaking required)

2 c almonds, soaked
1 c cashews, soaked
1 T fresh-squeezed lemon juice
1/5 c dulse flakes
½ tsp sea salt
2 stalks celery, minced
1/8 red onion, minced
¾ c filtered water (as needed)

1) Soak Almonds + Cashews separately overnight, rinse + drain.
2) Pulse/ chop almonds in the food processor until coarsely chopped, then place in a mixing bowl.
3) To make cashew mayo, blend cashew, lemon, salt + ¾ cup water until smooth, creamy, + delicious! Pour over chopped almonds in mixing bowl.
4) Mince celery + onion (finely chopped) + add to bowl.
5) Add dulse flakes, stir till mixed well, + eat! Absolutely delicious!!

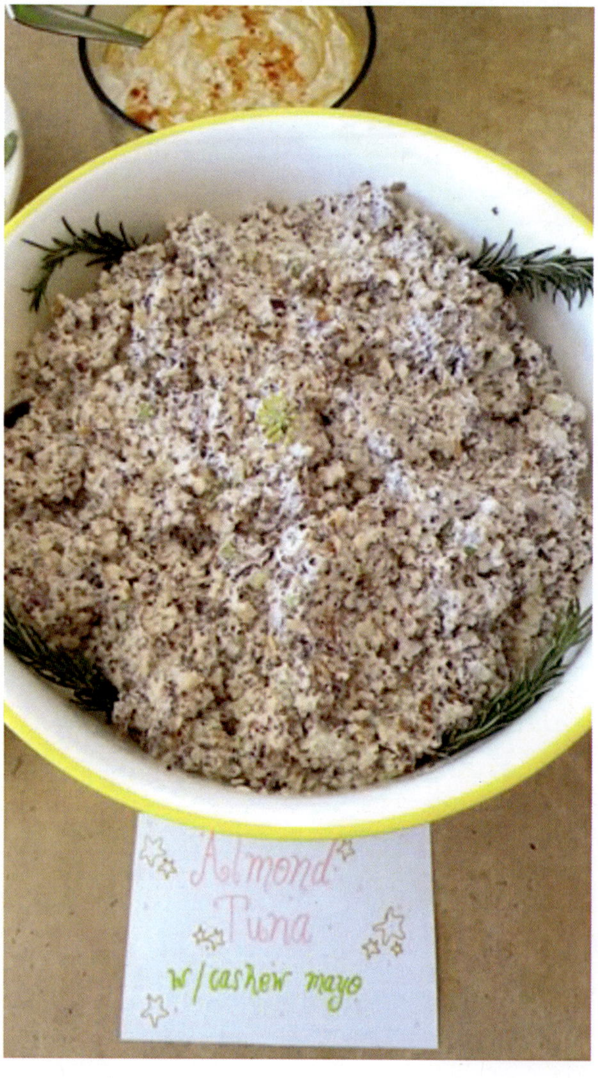

♥Carrot-Raisin Salad

Serves: 10-12
Time: 15 minutes (requires overnight soaking)

1 lb carrots, shredded
1 cup raisins, soaked
2 T fresh-squeezed orange juice
3 T fresh squeezed lemon juice
1 tsp cinnamon
pinch sea salt
2 T raw local honey

1) Wash carrots, then grate/ shred in the food processor, add to mixing bowl.
2) Add soaked raisins to the bowl (soak overnight in filtered water just enough to cover raisins). The next morning, drain water (you can save raisin water to use as a sweetener in other recipes ;)).
3) Add all other ingredients, including raw local honey to sweeten! Enjoy!! (Adjust to taste! You are welcome to add fresh mint, fresh fennel/ fennel seeds, or other ingredients that suit your fancy!)

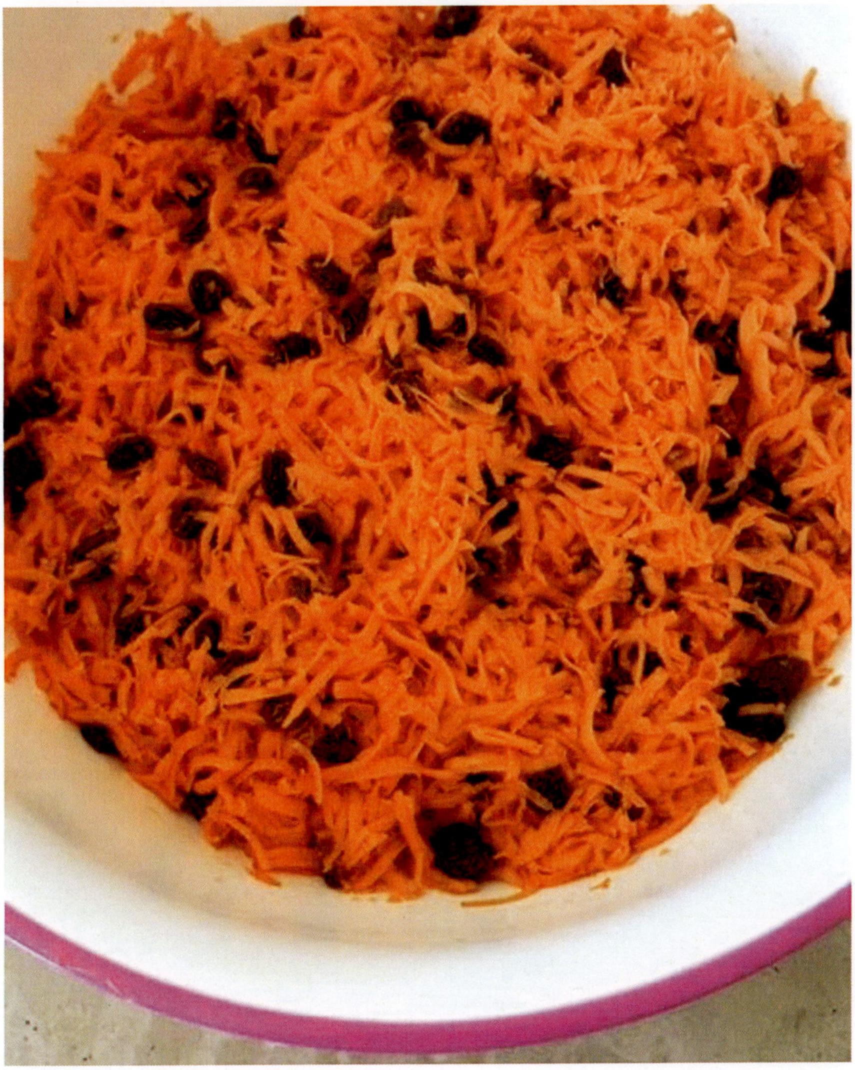

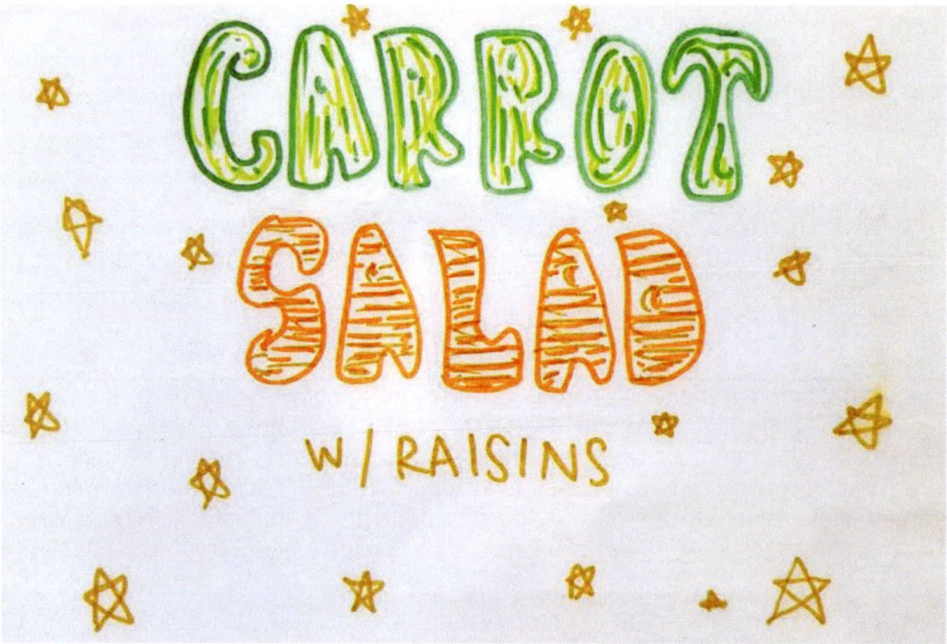
CARROT
SALAD
W/ RAISINS

♥∆Seaweed Salad
Serves: 8
Time: 15 minutes (requires overnight soaking)

½ pack Wakame, soaked
1 small head pak choi, sliced thin into ribbons
4 T brown sesame seeds
3 T sesame oil
1 T fresh-squeezed lime juice
3 green onions, thinly sliced

1) Cover seaweed overnight to soak. Drain water, if any is left, + add to mixing bowl.
2) Chop bok choi + green onions finely, add to seaweed.
3) Add all other ingredients, stir + enjoy!!

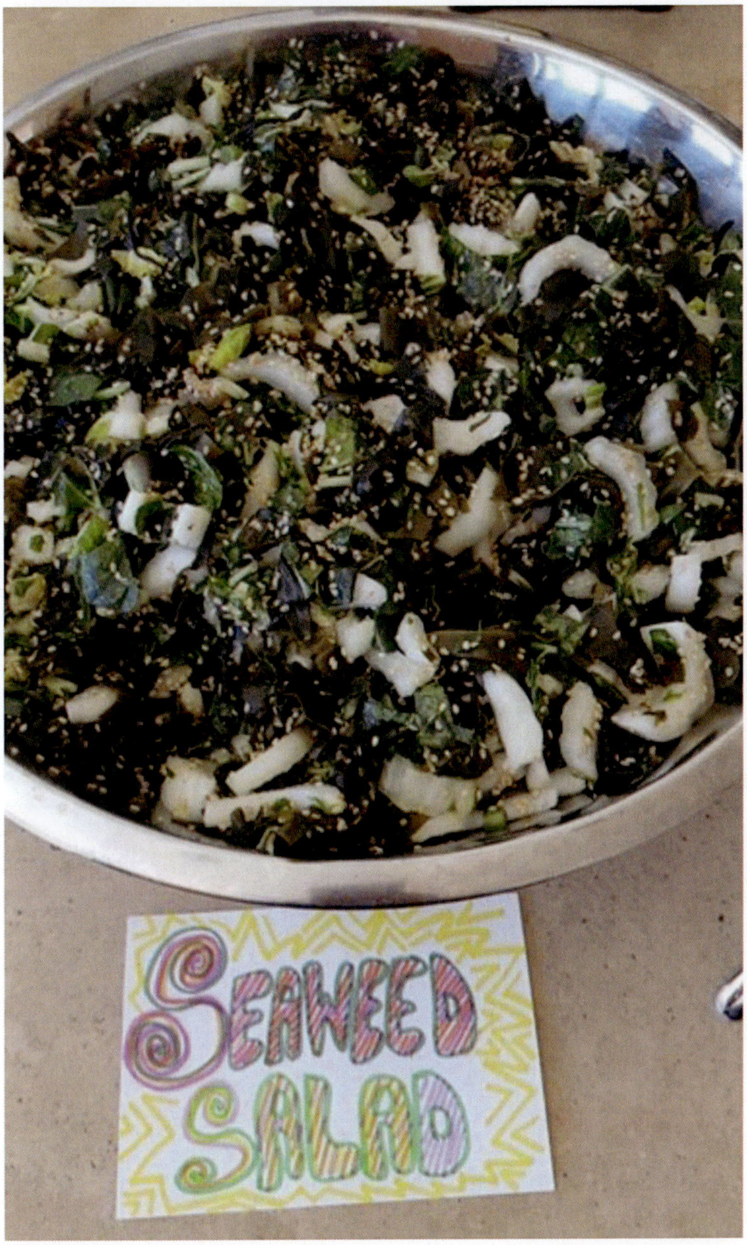

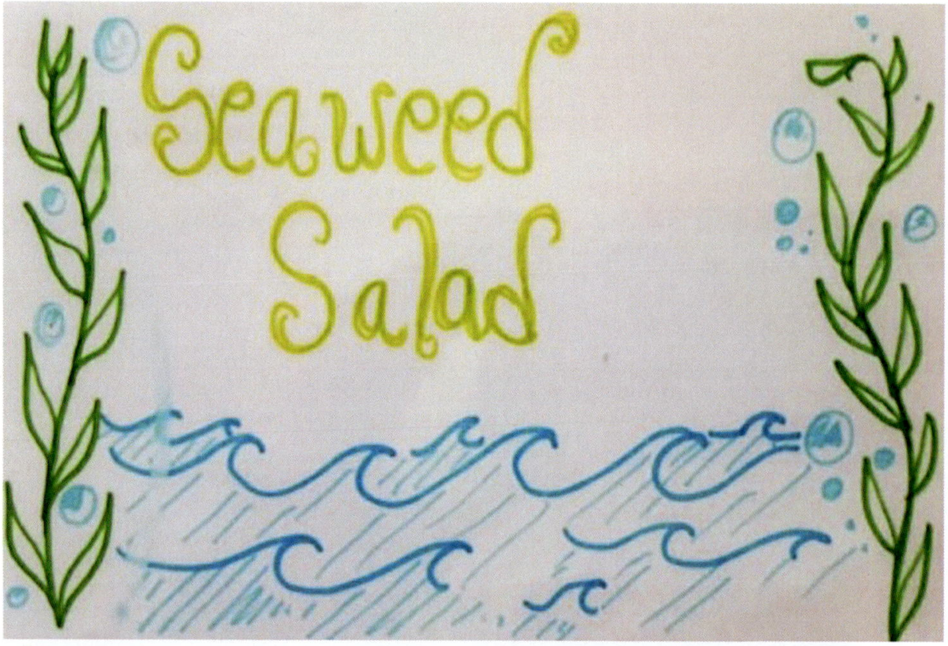
Seaweed
Salad

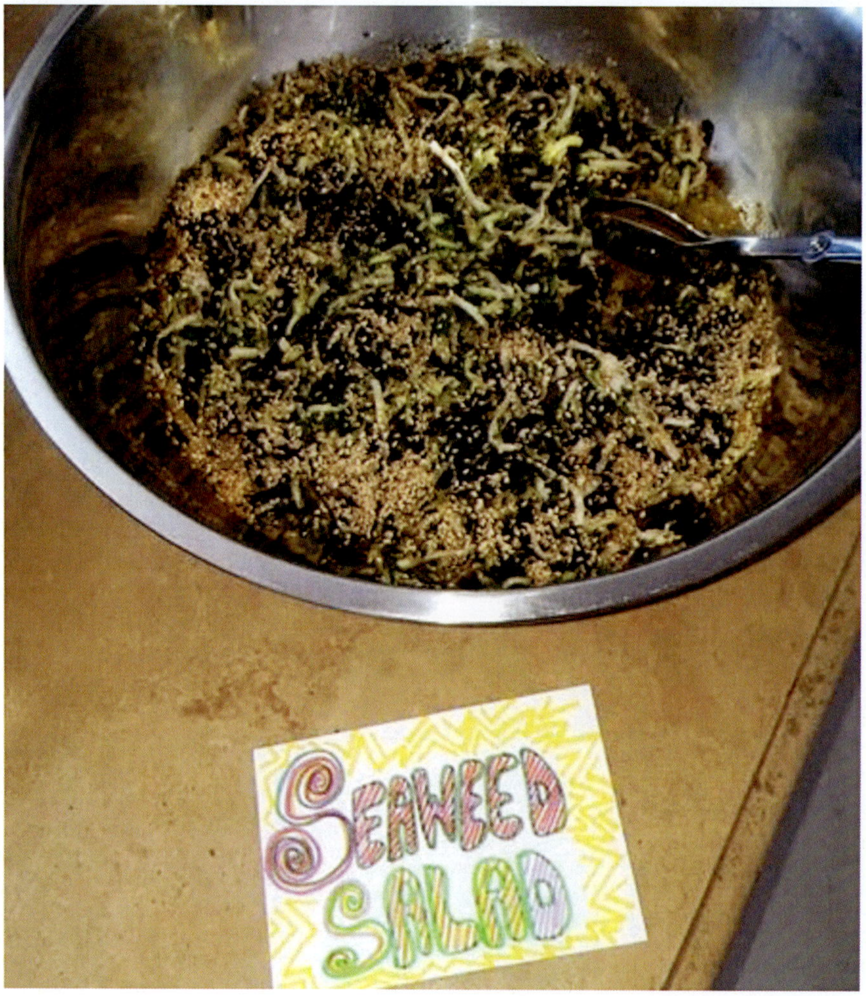
SEAWEED
SALAD

Roasted Beets/ Cauliflower/ Roots
Serves: 8
Time: 45 minutes

4 beets, cut into bite-size "chunks"
1 head cauliflower, cut into "chunks"
2 yellow potatoes, cut into "chunks"
7 carrots (or 8! ;)), cut into "chunks"
2 sprigs fresh rosemary, de-stemmed
2 T olive oil
1 tsp sea salt

1) Cut roots + cauliflower into chunks. Place into a mixing bowl. Add fresh rosemary.
2) Toss w/ olive oil + sea salt, making sure all veggies are coated!
3) Bake @ 350 degrees on an olive-oiled baking pan/ or glass dish.
4) When kitchen starts smelling great, check w/ fork to see if they are done!
5) Enjoy! This is a great dish to add to the Salad Bar!! ;)

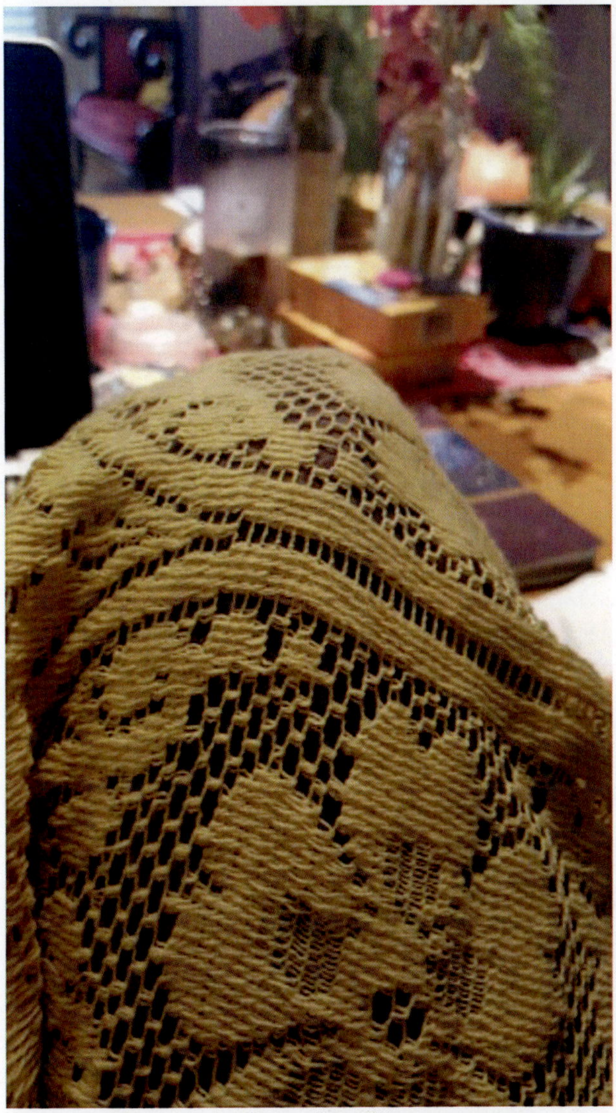

kitchen table altar/ pondering the writing process ♥

⊕Hard-Boiled Eggs

Serves: 24
Time: 30 minutes

1 dozen free-range, pastured organic local eggs (the kind with dark orange yolks!)
water for boiling
pinch sea salt

1) Place eggs in a single layer at the bottom of a big pot. Cover with water, 2 inches above egg level. ;) Add a pinch of sea salt.
2) Turn stove on high + bring the water to a boil.
3) Once water is boiling, turn off the heat, cover with lid, + let sit for 10-12 minutes.
4) Carefully pour off water from the pot (using the lid to protect eggs), + run cool water over the eggs to stop the cooking process.
5) Peel eggs, using water/ running water to help the process be easy!
6) Cut each hard-boiled egg in half + arrange on a tray to serve!

A note about eggs: I went vegetarian in high school because meat grossed me out, when I thought about what it actually was + where it was from. I never knew you could even *be* vegetarian, until I made my first vegetarian friend, Meredith, while working at Jewish summer camp in 1995! (I would otherwise, just cry at the dinner table when chicken was served on the bone. ;))

In 2000, after writing a Philosophy paper on Animal Rights in college, I decided to become vegan. Partially because I believed animals were not here for human pleasure, but because of their own life, which is valid in its own right! And a big reason was the system of factory farming. I'm sure you've seen some of the documentary films, + they are deeply disturbing.

However, years later, visiting small farms + neighbors' backyards where they keep chickens, does not bother me morally. I worked at the Local Farmstand in Atlanta in 2006/7, where we sold eggs from Crystal Organic Farm, + I decided to try them myself. I would make omelettes with squash blossoms + local greens, + eat them with my green smoothies or acai. Add to the fact that my body was craving eggs, + I feel way more emotionally stable with the Vitamin K + a lil bit of animal protein. And I really do love eggs!

I am not one of those people who will just eat eggs in a restaurant. They need to be organic, or free-range, for me to say yes. I seek out brunch places that serve organic eggs. Or I cook them myself at home. The best eggs I have ever had come from small local farms or a neighbor's backyard. If it resonates, try it yourself! Don't "buy into" the system of factory farming. Eat with your conscience, everything is energy!! Ask a restaurant where they get their eggs from, + put in a request for organic/ free-range/ pastured eggs. And don't order them until they change their sourcing! We can change the world with our wallets! ;)

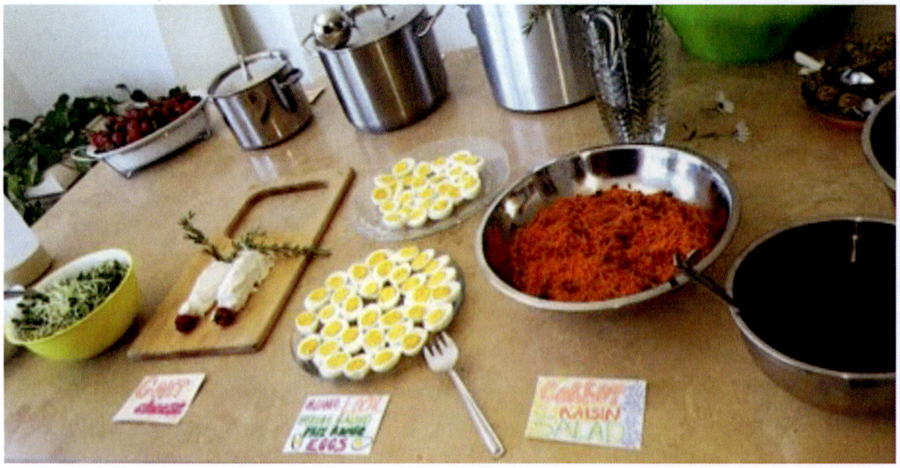

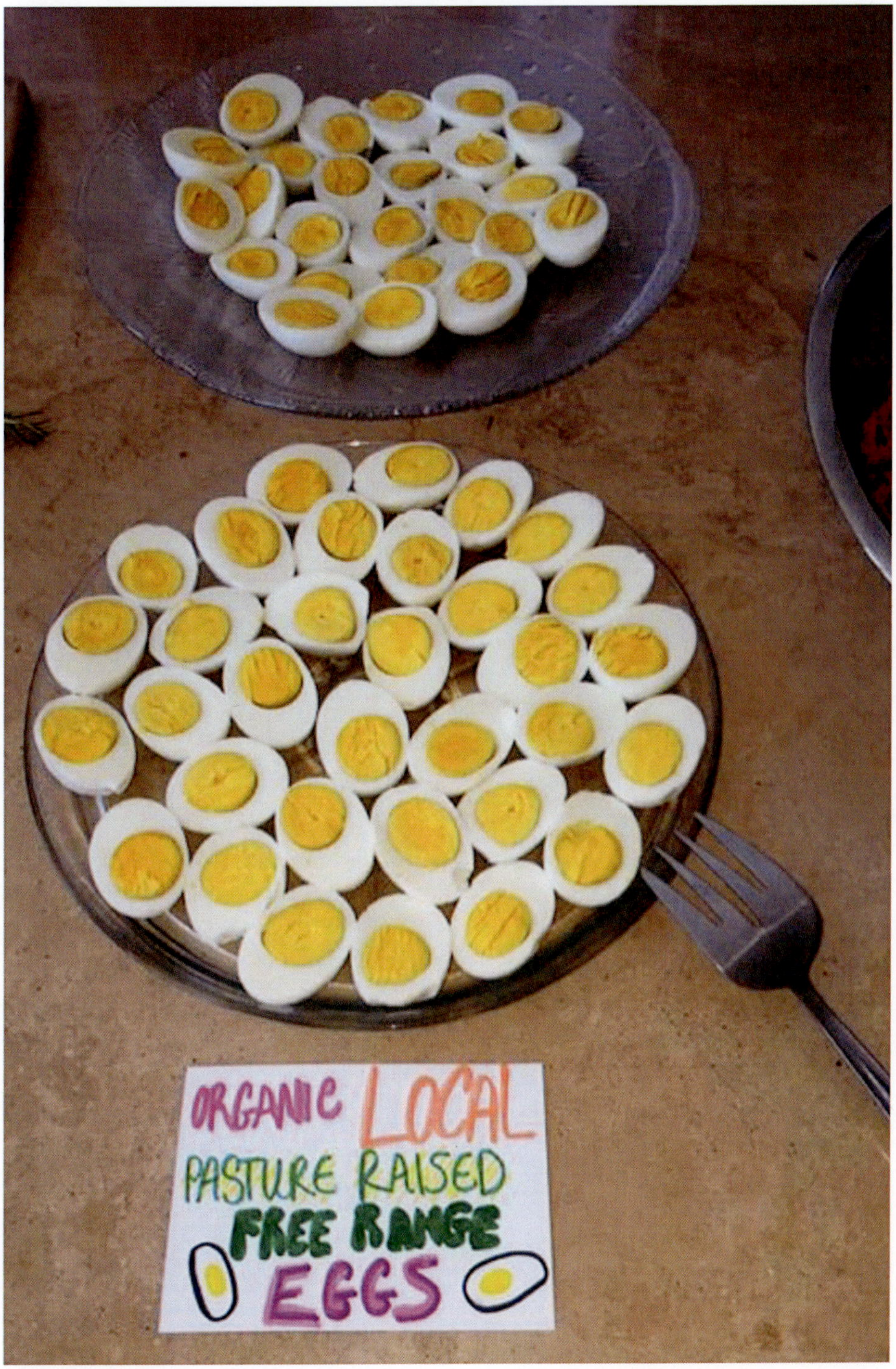
ORGANIC LOCAL
PASTURE RAISED
FREE RANGE
EGGS

♥∆Cashew Coconut Whipped Crème: A Raw/ Cooked Vegan Fusion
Serves: 4
Time: 15 minutes (requires overnight soaking)

1 c Cashews, soaked
1 can Coconut Milk
1/3 c Raw Local Honey
1 t vanilla extract
pinch sea salt
filtered water (as needed)

1) Soak cashews overnight. Drain + rinse.
2) Put all ingredients into blender, except filtered water. Blend using tamper/ plunger to help mix whipped crème. Add water, only if needed to thin out the consistency.
3) Eat with fresh, local strawberries!! Yum Yum!!!

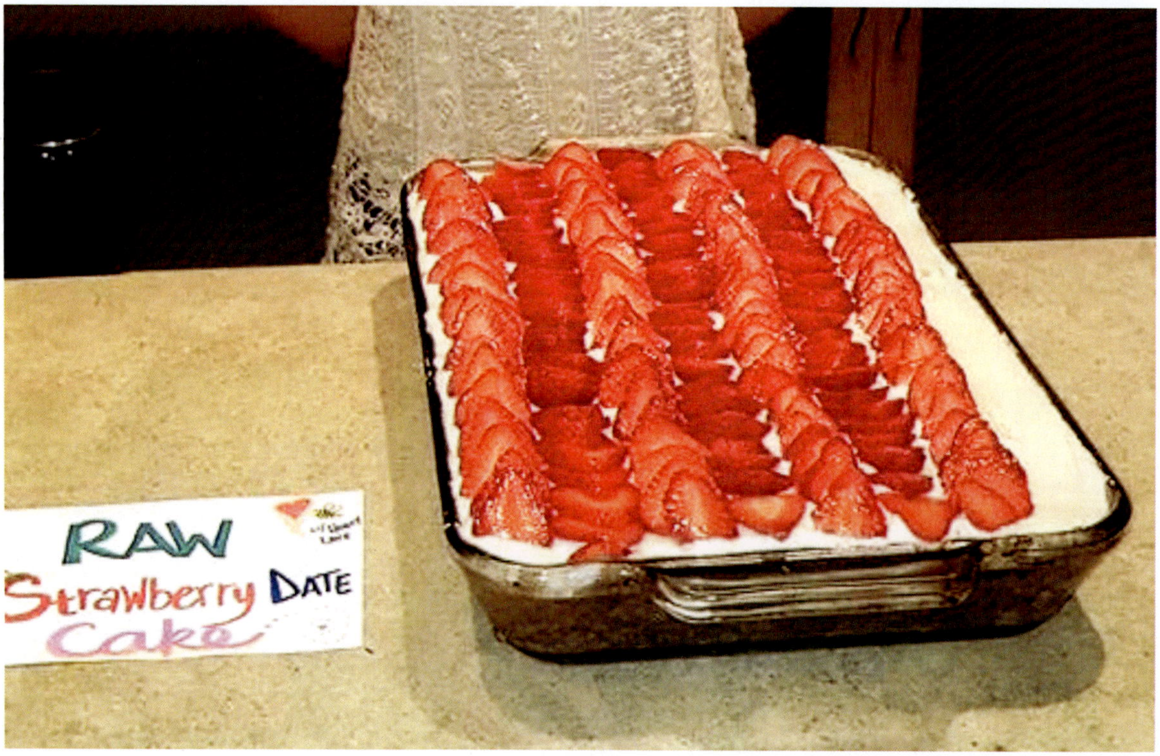

Thai Curry Dinner

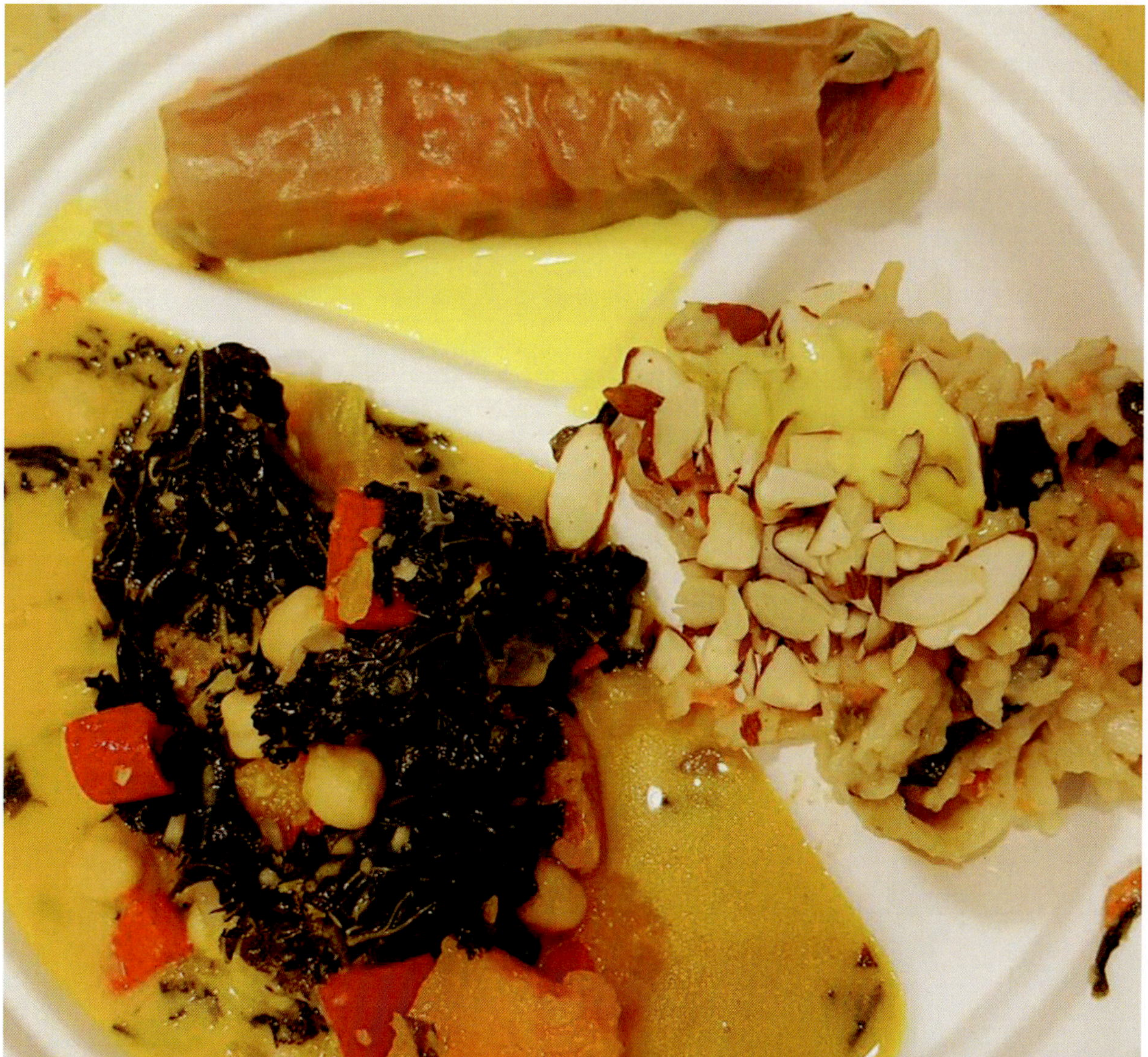

ΔThai Coconut Curry w/ Summer Squash, Chickpea, Vegetables
Serves: 4
Time: 90 minutes

1 cup chickpeas, cooked
1 T coconut oil
1 small yellow onion, diced
1 T ginger, minced/ chopped finely
2 cloves garlic, minced/ pressed
1 red bell pepper, diced
1 c yellow summer squash, cut into small-medium "chunks"
2 T Thai red curry paste (be sure to buy a brand without sugar… I like "Thai Kitchen" brand)
1 can coconut milk
½ bunch kale, washed + chopped in thin ribbons
1 tsp Grade B maple syrup
2 tsp Bragg's liquid aminos
1 ½ tsp rice vinegar
¼ bunch basil
¼ bunch cilantro

1) Soak chickpeas overnight w/ filtered water. Use 2-3 times as much water as chickpeas, as they will expand to soak up all the water!
2) The next day, drain water from chickpeas, + rinse 2-3 times with running water, to remove any residue + keep the beans fresh + easily digestible! Ideally the 3rd time, the water will run clear + they are ready to cook!
3) Cook chickpeas in filtered water (again, twice as much water as split peas) along with a pinch of sea salt/ pink Himalayan salt.
4) Meanwhile in a separate pan, heat up coconut oil + sauté chopped onion, pressed garlic, finely chopped ginger. Heat until the onion is clear.
5) Add sautéed ingredients + yellow squash to chickpea pot. Bring to a boil.
6) Once pot is boiling, take heat down to low. Add kale, cilantro, basil, + all other ingredients. Continue to cook on low heat until chickpeas are soft (up to 1 hour).

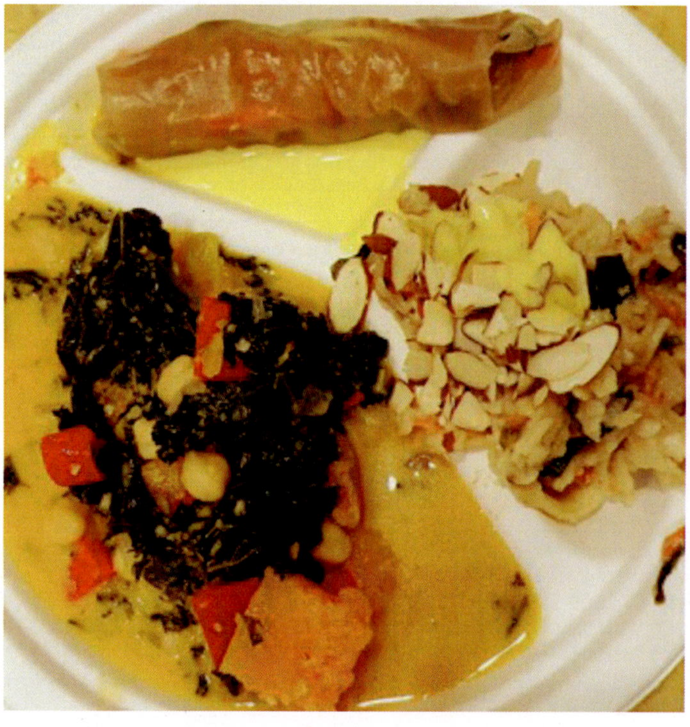

♥Brown Rice Paper Spring Rolls

Serves: 10 (1 roll each)
Time: 30 minutes

A special thanks to Kim Huynh for the Spring Roll inspiration… we spent many a hot summer day in ATL enjoying a version of these! I appreciate you sharing your "Healthy Vietnamese" version with me! ;)

10 brown rice spring roll wrappers (I like Star Anise Foods brand)
10 leaves leafy green lettuce
1 large cucumber
2 large carrots
1 large avocado
½ bunch fresh basil
1 large mango
2 T hot pepper sesame oil
2 tsp sea salt
6 T brown sesame seeds

1) Cut cucumber, mango, carrot, + avocado into "matchstick" slices.
2) Wash + pull basil leaves off stem. Wash lettuce leaves.
3) Mix together in a small bowl: hot pepper sesame oil, sea salt, + brown sesame seeds.
4) Soften brown rice paper in a flat dish with lukewarm water, then layer lettuce leaf, cucumber, carrots, avocado, mango, basil, + a dollop of sesame seed mixture. Fold bottom of rice paper up, then fold 2 sides in, then roll bottom towards the top. Lay rice paper roll flap side down to set.
5) Repeat with other rice paper rolls.
6) Eat + enjoy!

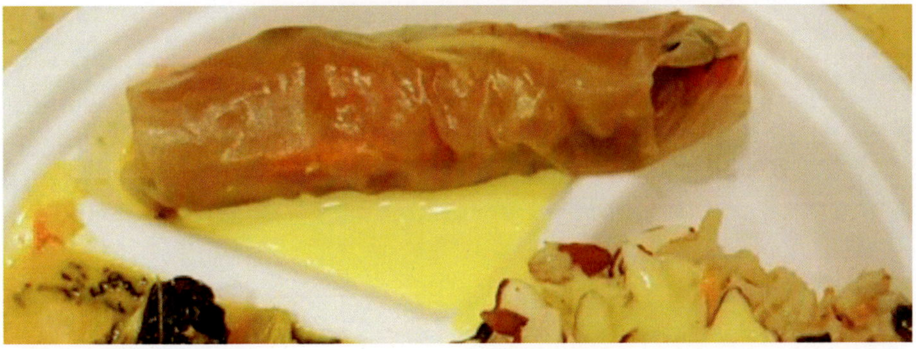

ΔPlain Brown Rice for Curry
Serves: 6
Time: 1 hour (also requires overnight soaking)

1 cup dry Brown Rice (= 3 cups cooked)
pinch Sea Salt
Filtered Water

1) Soak rice overnight. Drain + rinse.
2) Cook 1 part soaked rice to 1 ½ parts water. Add a pinch of sea salt. (Would normally be 1 part rice to 2 parts water, but rice has expanded from soaking. ;))
3) Bring water to a boil (high heat), then turn down to low + simmer until rice is cooked all the way (about 45 minutes).

♥Green Salad
Serves: 4
Time: 15 minutes

1 head green/ red leaf lettuce, washed + broken into bite-size pieces
½ cucumber, thinly sliced into rounds
½ container Sunflower Sprouts

1) Arrange lettuce in a circular salad bowl.
2) Decorate with cucumber slices + sunflower sprouts in a mandala around the edges of the bowl.
3) Enjoy with Cashew Ranch/ or other leftover dressing! Simple + Easy!

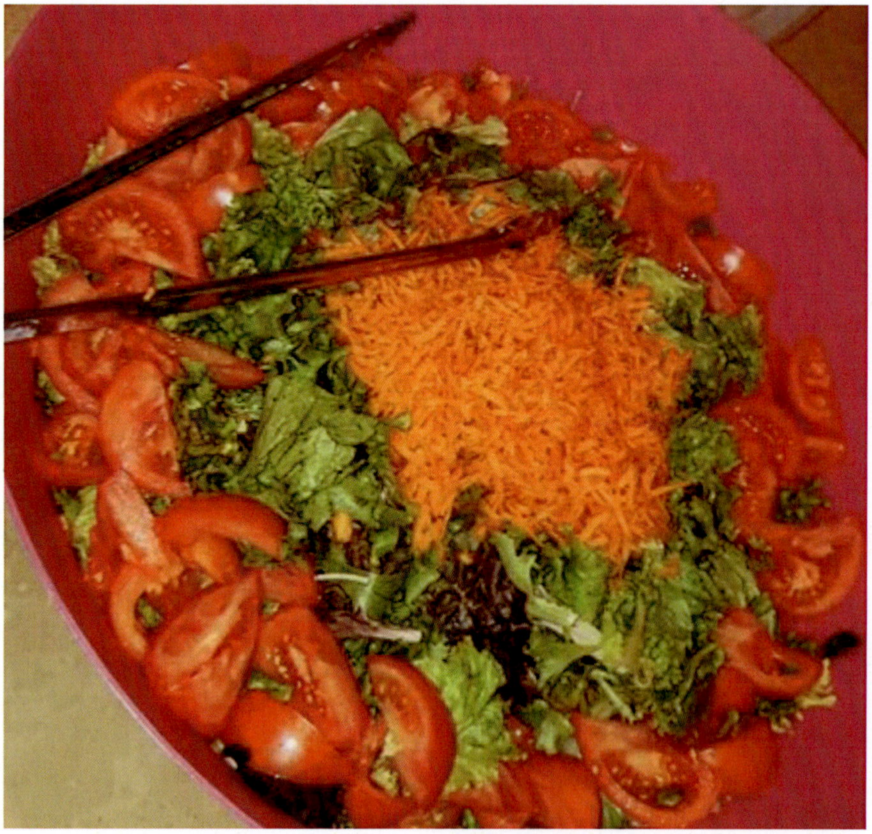

♥Raw Vegan Brownie Bites – inspired by Minimalist Baker's No Bake Vegan Brownies with Chocolate Ganache, MinimalistBaker.com
Serves: 12
Time: 1 hour

1 cup Almonds, raw dry
1 cup Walnuts, raw dry
2 ½ cup Dates, pitted
¾ cup cacao powder
¼ tsp Sea Salt
1 t vanilla extract

Frosting (optional):

2/3 c cacao powder
1/3 c cacao butter
½ c raw local honey
2 T coconut oil
¼ tsp sea salt

1) In food processor, process walnuts + almonds until finely ground.
2) Add cacao powder + sea salt + pulse in food processor. Transfer everything to mixing bowl.
3) Process pitted dates until chopped + smooth as possible. Put chopped dates in a second bowl.
4) Add nut mixture back into blender, + add date mixture little by little until totally smooth.
5) Press "brownie batter" into a non-stick or coconut oil-greased pan, until even + can be eventually cut into squares.
6) For frosting, melt cacao butter + coconut oil in a double boiler or in a bowl in the dehydrator. Then blend all frosting ingredients together in the Vitamix.
7) Pour frosting over brownie pan, then set in freezer for 20 minutes to chill.
8) Score + cut brownies, eat + enjoy!!!

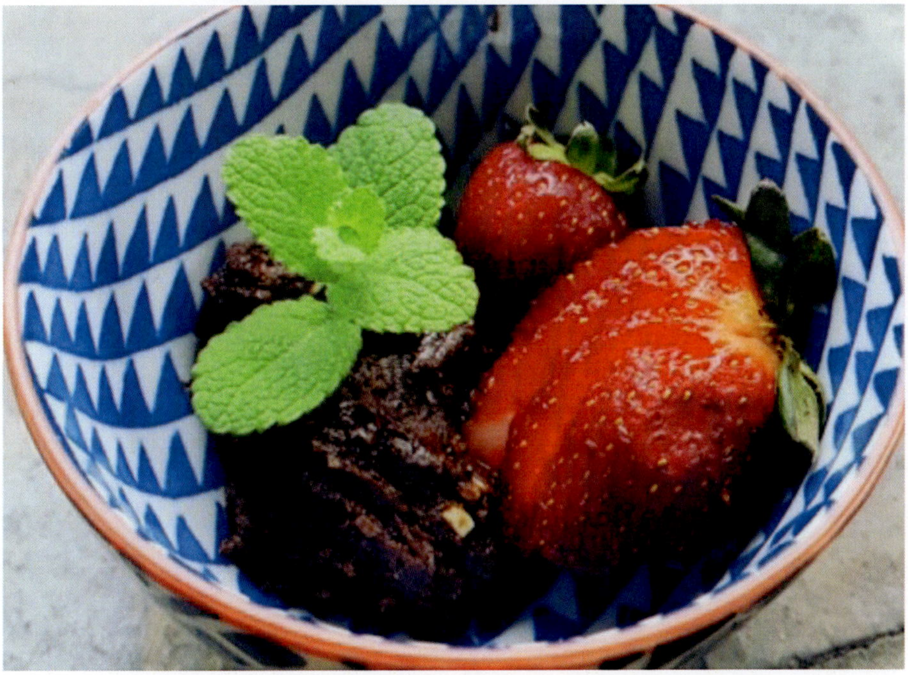

Pizza Lunch

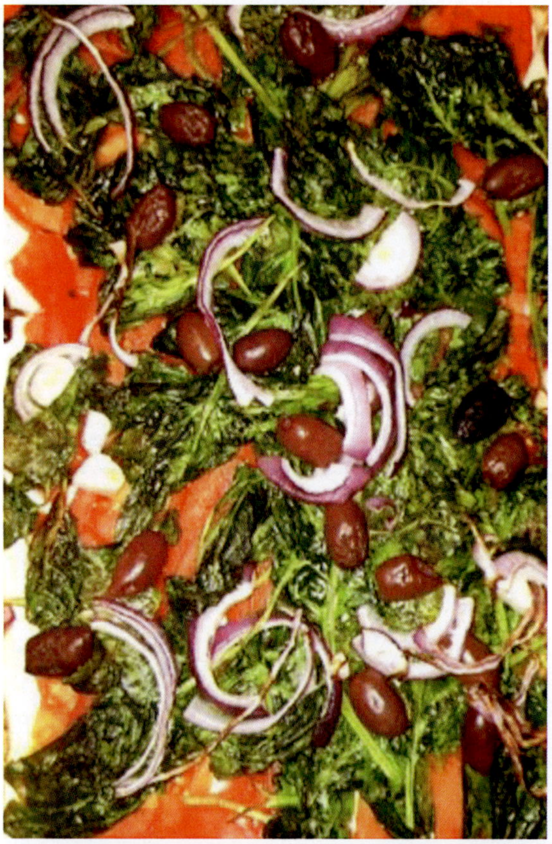

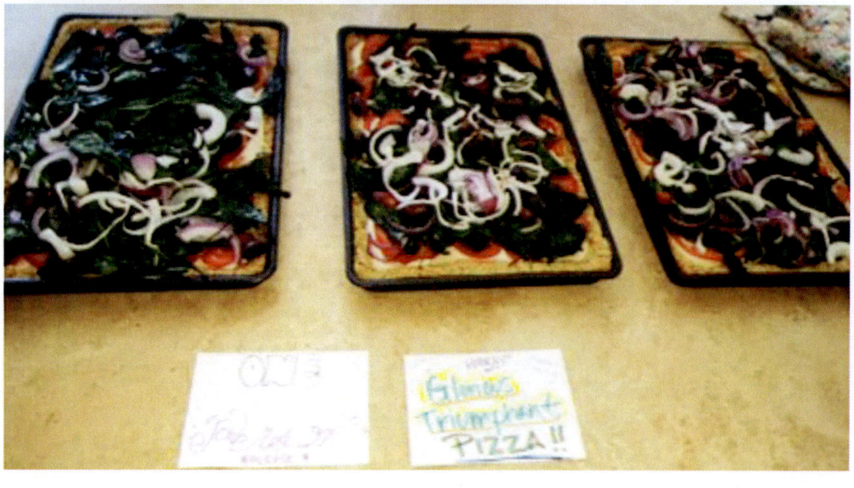

∆Gluten-Free Oat Groat-Cauliflower Crust Pizza w/ Tomato, Spinach, Olive, Onion, + Cashew Cheese!

Serves: 4
Time: 1 ½ hours

Crust:
1 c oat groats, soaked
1 c cauliflower, pulsed in food processor
1 T ground flax (optional)
2 sprigs fresh rosemary
1 tsp olive oil
1/3 tsp sea salt

Toppings:
1 ½ tomatoes
½ bunch spinach
1 T olive oil for marinating spinach
½ sweet onion
½ cup Kalamata Olives (or pitted Olives of choice! ;))
¼ bunch basil

Cashew Cheese:
1 ½ c soaked raw cashews
½ c filtered water
2 T lemon juice
½ tsp sea salt

1) Soak oat groats overnight, then drain + rinse. In a separate container, also soak cashews for cheese overnight, then drain + rinse as well. ;)
2) Pulse cauliflower till fine, in the food processor, then transfer to bowl.
3) Process Fresh Rosemary first in the food processor till chopped, then add oat groats + process. Finally, add cauliflower. Add olive oil + sea salt. Add filtered water if needed, to "turn" into a dough.
4) Line baking sheet w/ olive oil + shape crust onto the pan. You can do one big crust for everyone, or 4 mini-crusts. ;) It's fun to raise the crust up on the edges, like real pizza. ;)
5) Bake crust @ 350 degrees for 20 minutes.
6) Next, to make the cashew cheese, place all ingredients in the blender + blend. Add cheese to the top of baked pizza crust.
7) Next, wilt spinach in olive oil (toss/ marinate), slice tomatoes + onions finely, + pick fresh basil off the stem. Add all toppings, including olives, on top of the cheese.
8) Bake finished pizzas at 350 degrees for 20-30 minutes, or until light golden brown on the edges. Yum! Eat + Enjoy! Grab em' fast! They're gonna go! ;)

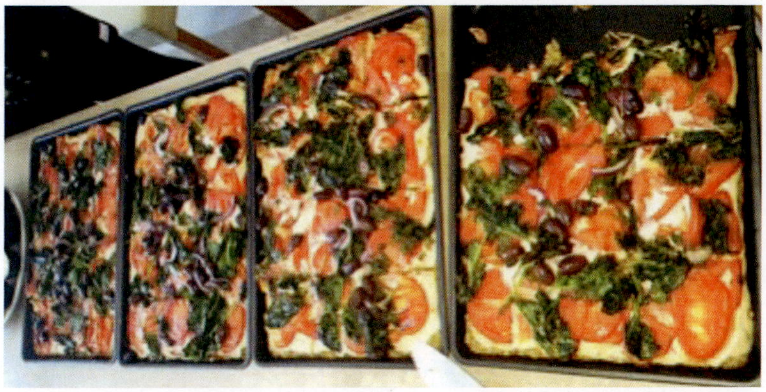

♥Green Salad w/ Ume Plum Vinaigrette
Serves: 4
Time: 20 minutes

1 head Leafy Green Lettuce, washed + cut into bite-size pieces
2 Avocados, sliced
2 Tomatoes, cut in "chunks"
2 c Sunflower Sprouts
1 large Cucumber, sliced into rounds, or cut into bite-size "chunks"
3 carrots, shredded in food processor
½ beet, shredded in food processor
2 T ume plum vinegar
2 T olive oil

1) Arrange lettuce in a circular salad bowl. Toss lettuce with ume plum vinegar + olive oil. (Alternatively, you can toss with all the ingredients below, instead of decorating ;)).
2) Decorate with avocado, tomato, cucumber slices, carrot, beet + sunflower sprouts in a mandala around the edges of the bowl.
3) Enjoy! Simple + Easy!

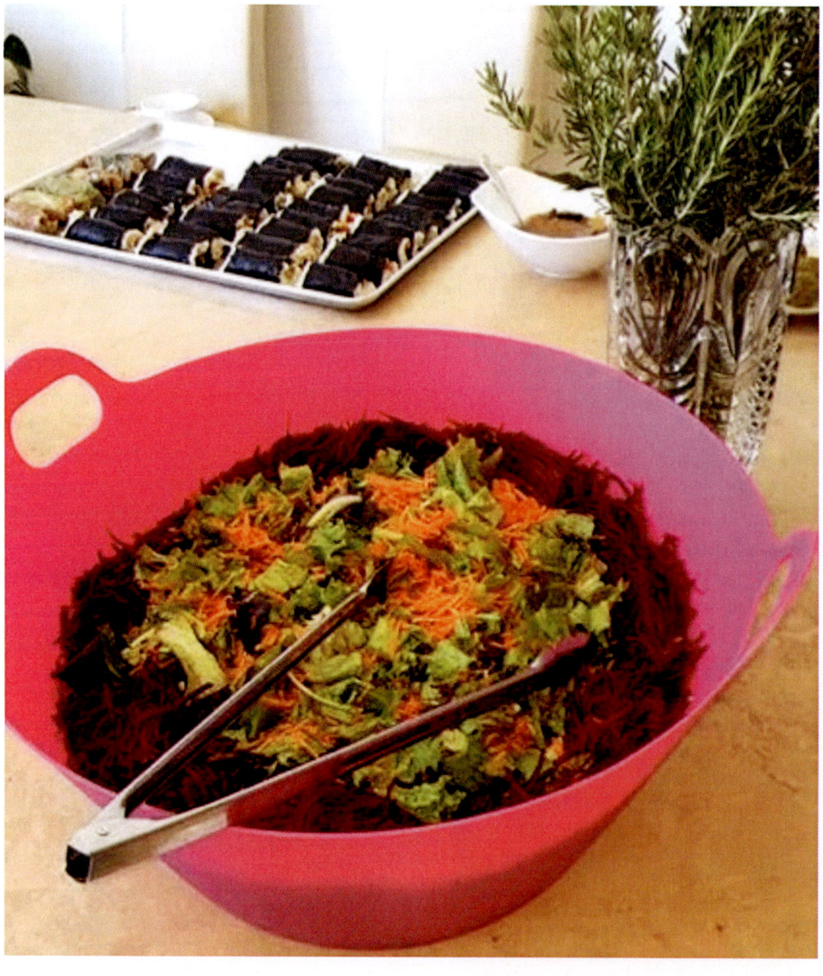

Buffalo Cauliflower Bites by Chef Julia Ahmadi (Julia is a Retreat Kitchen Goddess, but also an incredible classically-trained Chef, and incredible person!)
Serves: 4
Time: 30 minutes

This recipe is fun b/c it's gluten-free AND you get your protein from the chickpea flour! It's decadent comfort food, yet nothing is bad for you! ;) You can't go wrong! ;))

1 head Cauliflower
2/3 c chickpea flour (Bob's Red Mill is a good brand ;))
filtered water
1 tsp garlic powder
pinch cayenne
½ tsp sea salt
3 T coconut oil
1 fluid oz. Organic Hot Sauce (I love Melinda's brand Extra Hot Habanero, look for something with all-natural ingredients, no sugar!)
1 T Olive Oil

1) Cut Cauliflower into Floret "Chunks."
2) Mix chickpea flour, sea salt, garlic + cayenne. Then add filtered water to create a thick "batter" consistency.
3) Roll Cauliflower "chunks" into Chickpea batter.
4) Heat Coconut Oil in pan, then fry "Buffalo Cauliflower Bites" in coconut oil, turning to fry all sides.
5) Mix hot sauce + olive oil in a large mixing bowl.
6) Pour fried Buffalo Cauliflower Bites into hot sauce mixture + roll around/ coat.
7) Yum Yum! Eat up! These are not going to last! ;)) Enjoy!

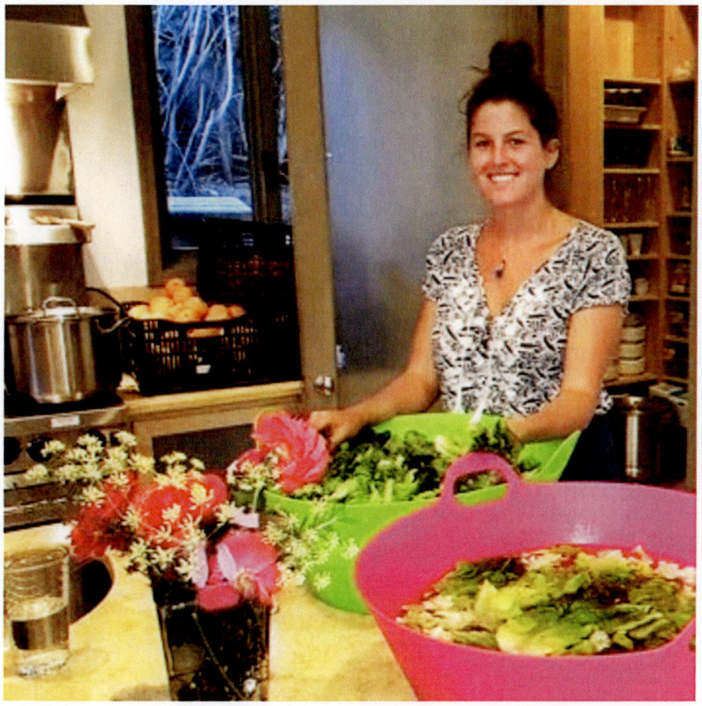

♥Chocolate Avocado Pudding (Raw!)

Serves: 3
Time: 15 minutes

1 Reed Avocado (large, if using Hass/ or smaller variety, use 2 Avocados)
½ c raw local honey
½ c raw cacao powder
1 tsp vanilla extract
1 pinch sea salt
¾ c filtered water

1) Cut Avocados in half + pit/ scoop avocado halves into the blender.
2) Add all other ingredients to blender.
3) Blend! Use tamper/ plunger to help pudding along.
4) Serve + enjoy!! People do not *believe* this is raw + healthy!! It tastes better than Jello pudding cups!!!! ;) You will WOW your guests!! ☺

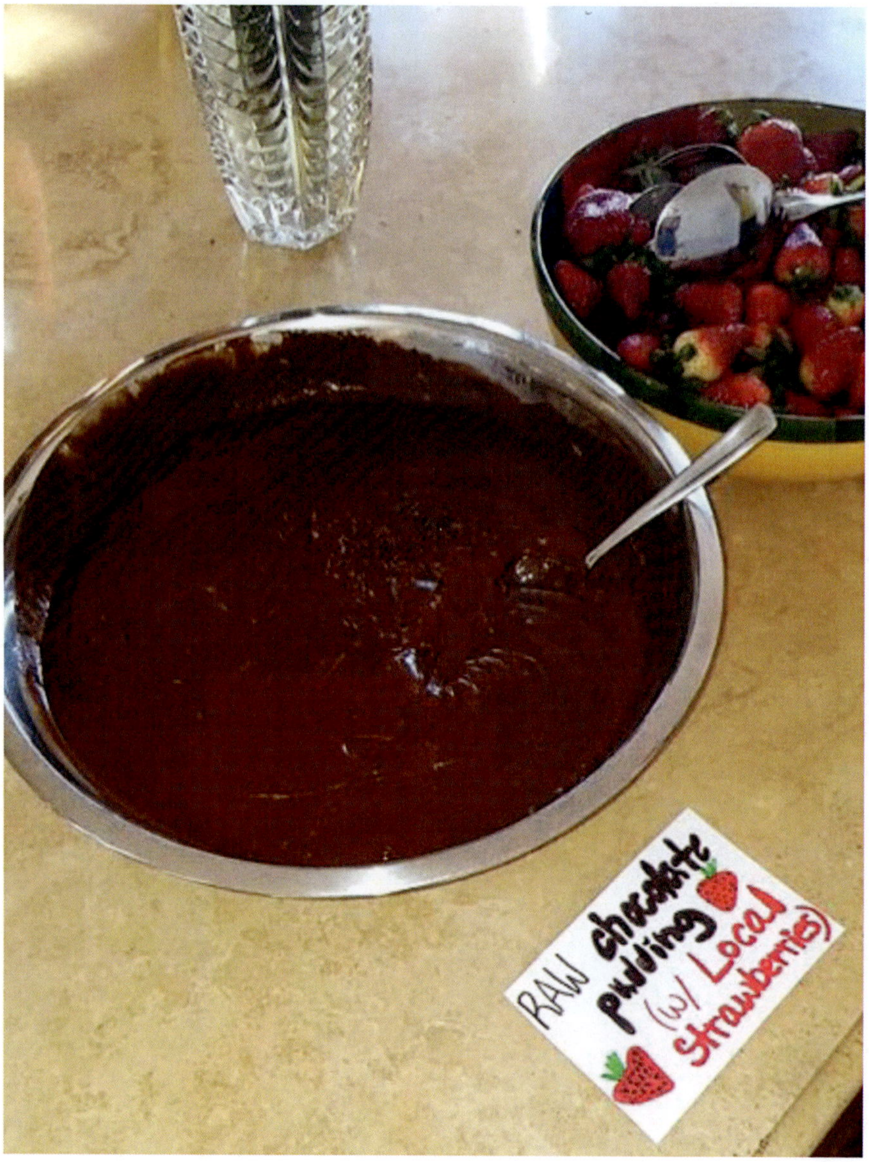

Pad Thai Night

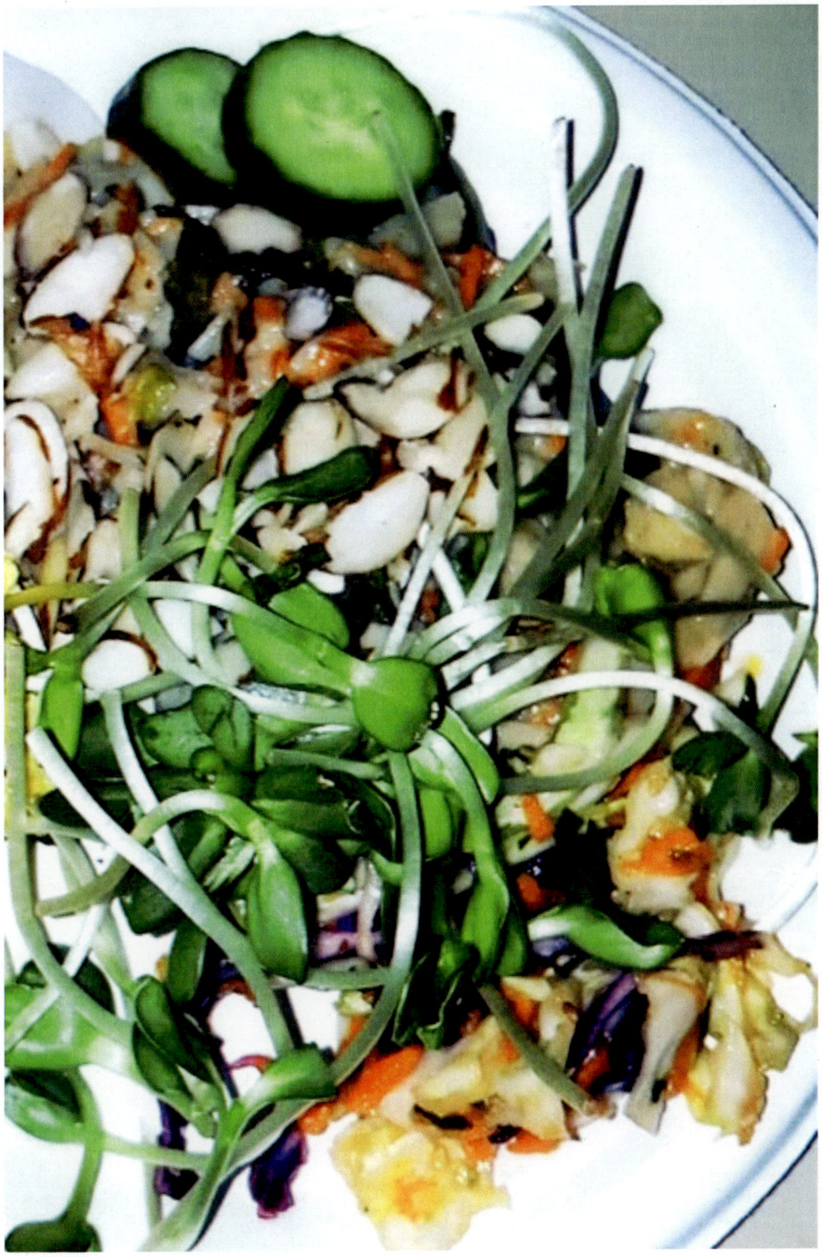

⊕Vegan (Vegetarian Optional) Pad Thai

Serves: 3
Time: 40 minutes

1 10-oz package rice noodles (I love Tinkyada brand gluten-free)
2 T olive oil
1 clove garlic
4 T Bragg's liquid aminos
2 T almond butter
2 limes
3 T raw honey/ or Grade B maple syrup
1 small red hot pepper
3 green onions, finely chopped (for garnish)
½ c chopped raw almonds (in food processor, for garnish)
1 head broccoli
½ package mung bean sprouts (the long white/ translucent kind)
1 grated carrot
½ cucumber (for garnish)
¼ bunch fresh basil
2 free-range organic eggs (optional)
2 small yellow squash, sautéed in olive oil (optional)

1) Finely chop green onions. Chop broccoli into "chunks." Chop/ pulse almonds in food processor until smaller, still crunchy pieces. Grate carrot using food processor. Slice cucumber into rounds. Save everything separately. Chop yellow squash into rounds + sauté in olive oil + garlic. Juice limes.
2) Boil water + cook noodles according to package stirring occasionally. Add broccoli to steam in cooking water with pasta at the very end – last few minutes.
3) While water is boiling, blend the Sauce: olive oil, Bragg's, almond butter, red hot pepper, maple syrup, lime juice + garlic.
4) When noodles are done, drain water, add sauce, carrots, green onions, + basil. Stir super well until everything is mixed together + all noodles are coated with the yummy goodness!
5) Serve with scrambled eggs cooked in coconut oil + sea salt on the side. Almonds on the side with a small serving spoon + sliced cucumbers on the side with serving fork.
6) Enjoy!!!

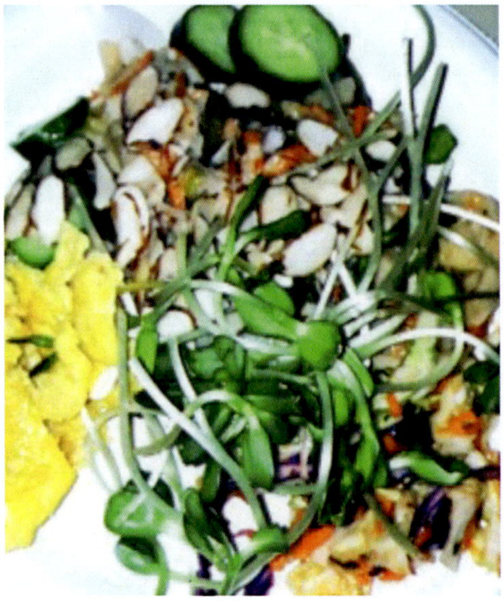

♥Green Salad w/ Avocado + Grapefruit Dressing

Serves: 4
Time: 10-15 minutes

Salad:

1 head Butter Lettuce, washed + cut/ ripped into bite-size pieces
1 Small Avocado, "chunked"
1 medium Grapefruit, sliced + peeled, with no inner skin, just the juicy part!

Dressing:

2 T olive oil
½ tsp sea salt
1 grapefruit, juiced

1) Arrange lettuce in a salad bowl.
2) Top with sprinkled avocado "chunks" + juicy grapefruit "chunks"
3) Blend dressing together in Vitamix, then pour over salad. Alternatively, pour/ sprinkle each ingredient separately over the salad. Then eat!! ☺ Refreshing + great for winter/ seasonal change.

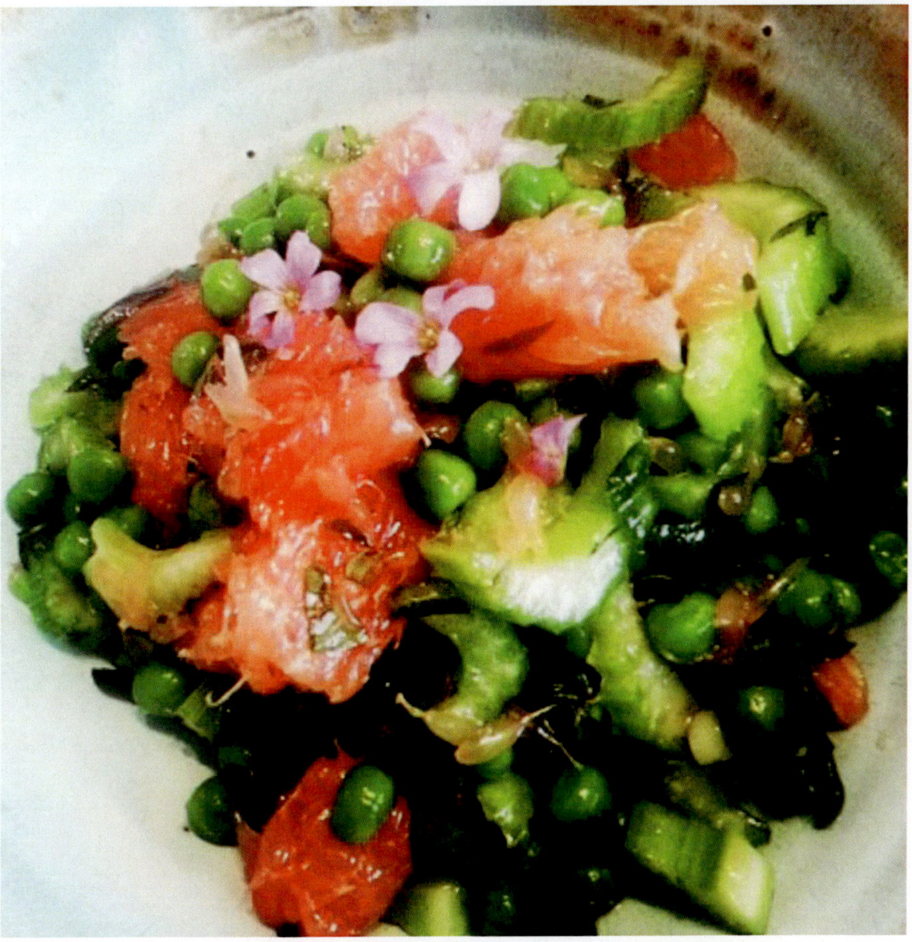

♥Cabbage-Carrot Slaw

Serves: 10 (this is a great one to save + use all week!)
Time: 15-20 minutes

1 large Green Cabbage, sliced thin
1/5 purple cabbage, sliced thin
5 carrots, shredded
½ c fresh-squeezed lime juice
1 T sea salt
1 T sesame oil (can be raw or toasted)
½ T hot pepper sesame oil
1 T grade B maple syrup
½ bunch cilantro, thinly chopped

1) Thinly slice cabbage + place in a large (stainless steel) mixing bowl.
2) Grate carrots in food processor + add to bowl.
3) Chop cilantro finely + add.
4) Add all other ingredients + stir!
5) This dish keeps really well! It's easy + yummy, + healthy!

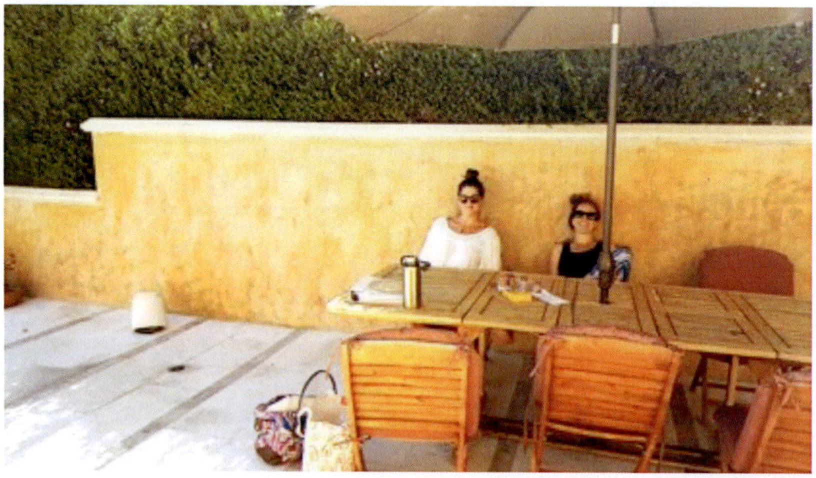

♥Mango Coconut Pudding

Serves: 4
Time: 40 minutes (10 minutes to make, 30 minutes to chill)

1 can coconut milk
¼ c chia seeds
2 T raw honey
½ tsp vanilla extract
½ fresh mango, peeled + cut from pit
pinch sea salt

1) Blend all ingredients (except for chia seeds) in the blender/ Vitamix.
2) Pour into a bowl/ container with cover, +stir in chia seeds until evenly mixed.
3) Allow to chill for 30 minutes in the fridge before eating.
4) Give one last stir to make sure the chia seeds are evenly mixed, serve + eat! You may top with additional mango chunks/ slices for decoration!

Veggie Burger Bar

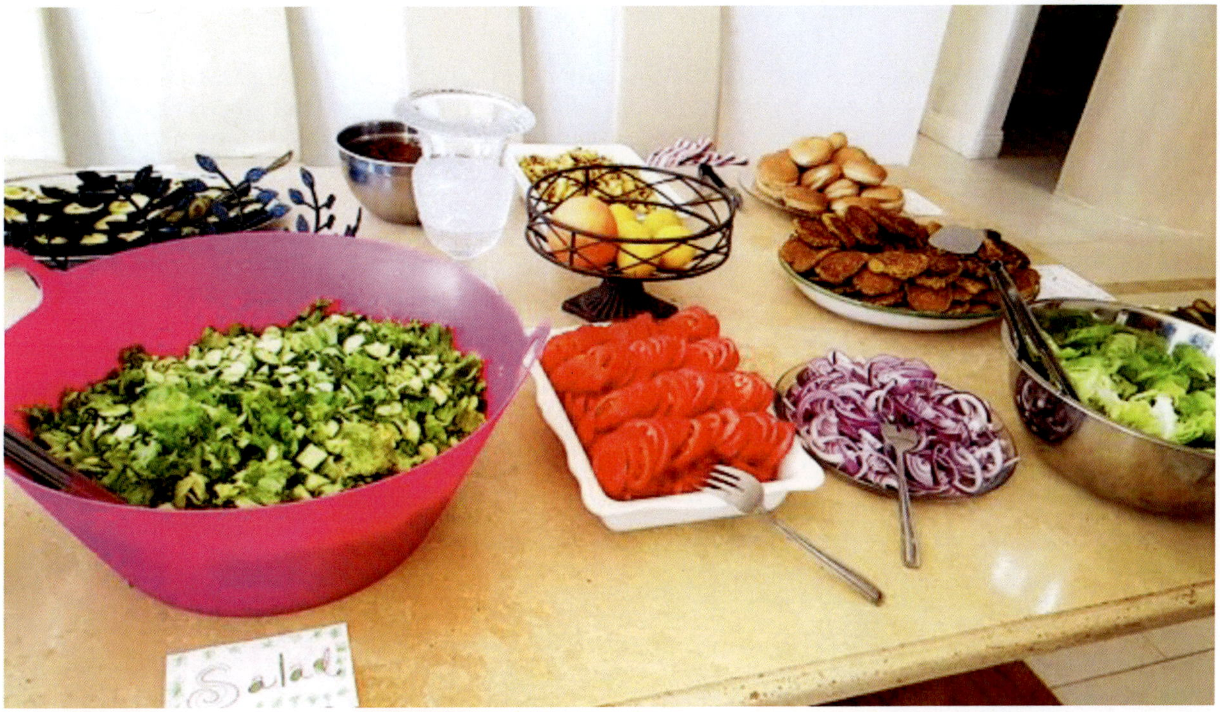

∇∆Lentil Burgers

Serves: 4
Time: 30 minutes (requires soaking lentils overnight, sprouting 1-2 days)

2 c soaked/ sprouted lentils (1 c dry lentil to start)
1 large carrot, chopped into "chunks"
1/3 c tomato, chopped into "chunks"
1 clove garlic
2 T olive oil
1 t sea salt
1 T cumin
1 t paprika
1 t dill
1 t coriander
pinch red pepper
1 t fresh-squeezed lemon juice
1 c chickpea flour (optional), as needed to bind together :)
1/3 c coconut oil (for frying)

1) Process in food processor first: garlic clove. Then add carrot + tomato chunks + process. Next add lentil sprouts + process till all ingredients are chopped. Next, add sea salt, olive oil, lemon juice, + spices + continue to process. Add chickpea flour if needed to bind burgers together.
2) Pour burger "batter" into a bowl, then roll + shape with hands into a ball, then flatten to make a burger patty.
3) Lightly fry burger patties in coconut oil, flipping when golden brown.
4) Serve with homemade ketchup recipe, sliced pickles, sliced onions, tomatoes + lettuce leaves. Add avocado slices + a gluten-free bun! (I've been using Ener-g Gluten-Free Hamburger Buns since they are vegan + sugar-free! I toast the buns, cut in half, in the oven for a few minutes before using ;)).
5) Note: Recipe can also be made using leftover beans, rice, quinoa, soup with liquid drained, etc. By simply adding the spices + chickpea flour, + frying! Eco-friendly + super Fun!

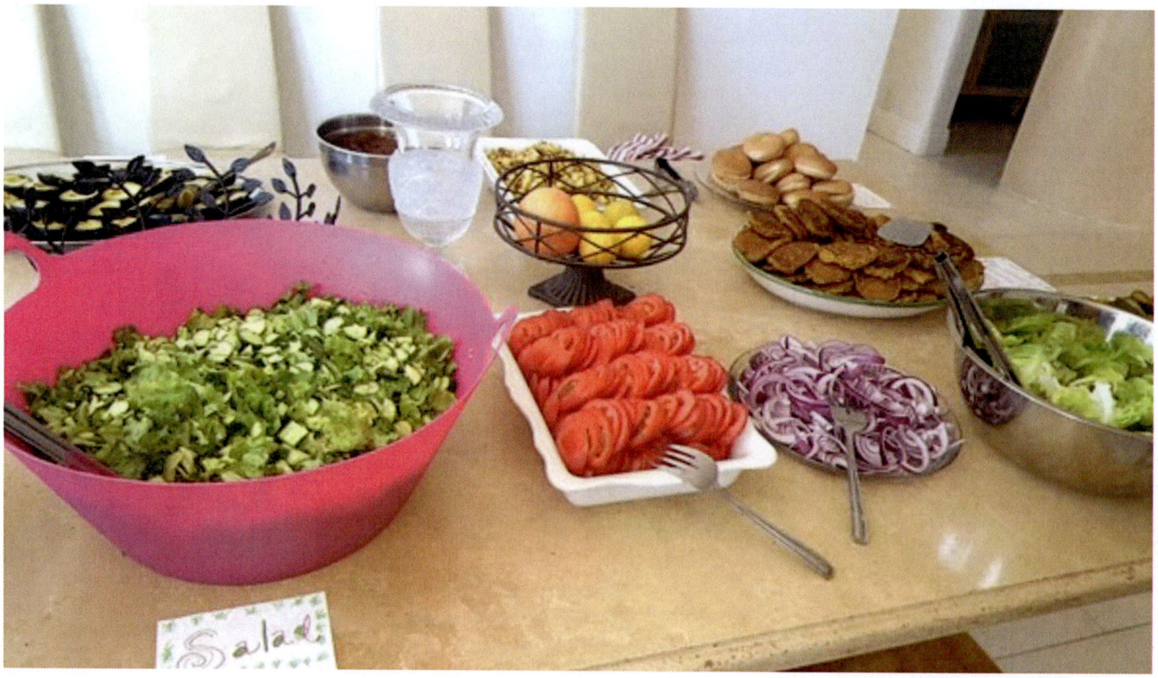

Burger Fixin's
Serves: 4
Time: 15 minutes

4 Bubbies Dill Pickles, sliced thin long ways
4-8 Lettuce Leaves, preferably fun + curly!
¼ red onion, sliced thin
1-2 tomatoes, sliced thin
1-2 avocados, sliced thin
4 Gluten-free Burger Buns (I've been using Ener-g Gluten-Free Hamburger Buns since they are vegan + sugar-free! I toast the buns, cut in half, in the oven for a few minutes before using ;)).

1) Wash, cut/ prep + serve all Burger Fixin's on a Serving Platter with Veggie Burgers + Buns! Top with Homemade Ketchup recipe + enjoy!!

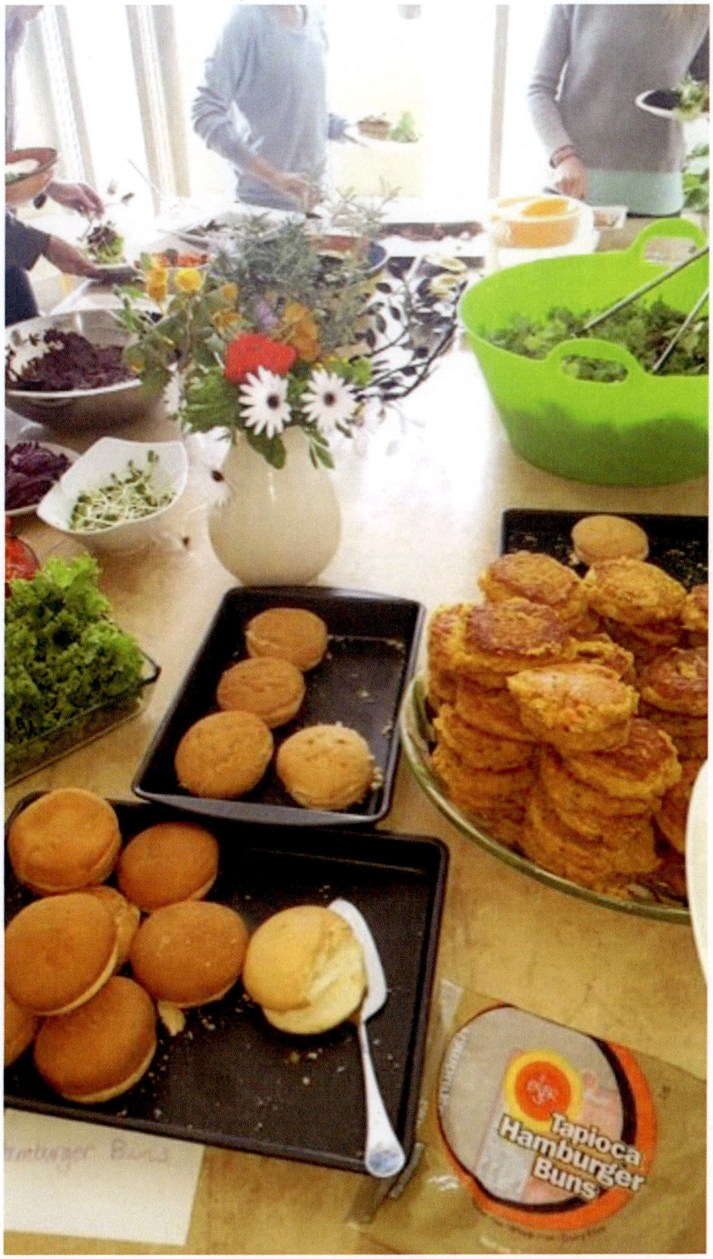

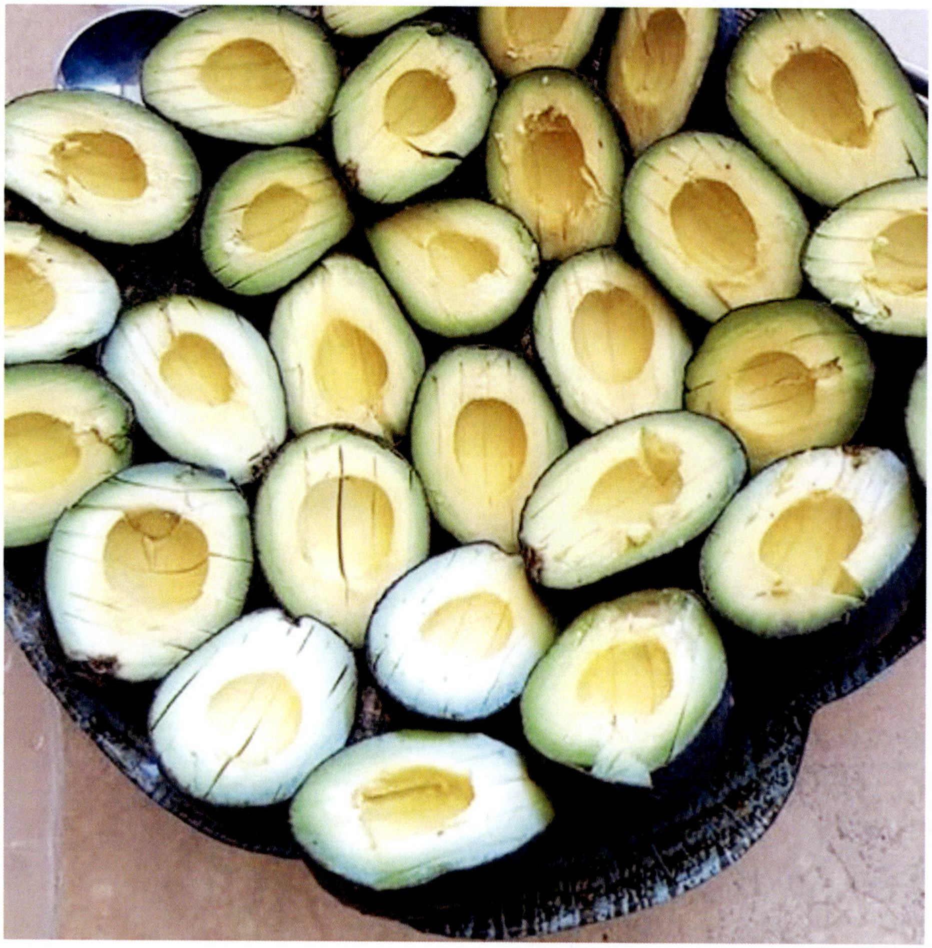

♥ΔRaw Vegan Basil Cashew Mayonnaise

Serves: 6
Time: 15 minutes (requires soaking cashews overnight)

1 ½ c soaked Cashews (1 c dry cashews, soaked overnight)
¼ c fresh-squeezed lemon juice
1 t sea salt
¼ c fresh Basil
1 T olive oil (optional)
water to desired consistency (1 ½ c)

1) Blend everything, except Basil, including filtered water, in blender/ Vitamix! Add the basil once the "Mayo" base is blended, to avoid the whole thing turning green, + rather, to have pretty basil "flecks." ;)
2) Yum Yum YUM! Enjoy!

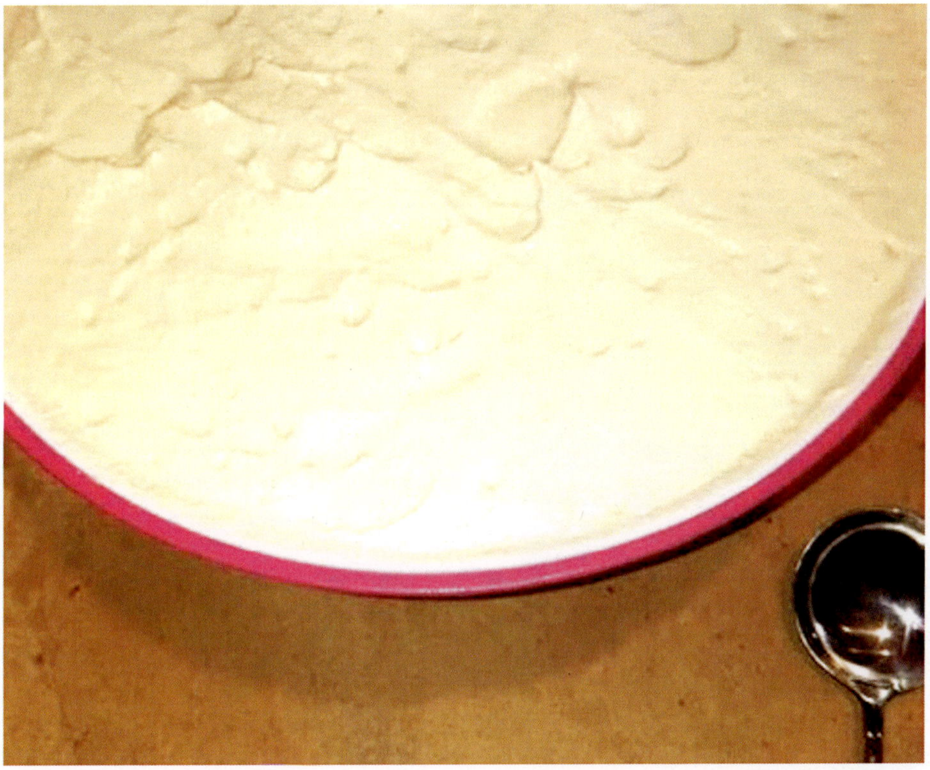

♥∆Raw Vegan Ketchup

Serves: 8
Time: 15 minutes (requires overnight soaking of sundried tomatoes)

1 c soaked Sundried Tomato (start w/ 2/3 c dry tomato, cover in water overnight, then drain water)
1 c fresh Tomato, cut into "chunks"
1 clove garlic
¼ c Onion
1 tsp Ginger
2 T Raw Local Honey/ or Grade B Maple Syrup
1 T apple cider vinegar (I like Bragg's brand – or one that still has the "Mother" vinegar culture flecks in the bottle – truly probiotic!)
½ t sea salt

1) Soak sundried tomato overnight (just barely covered in water). The next day, drain the water. (You can save + use for the liquid base of salad dressings + soups!)
2) Food process first: onion, ginger, garlic.
3) Then add fresh + sundried tomato, + process till evenly chopped.
4) Then add all other ingredients + process.
5) Adjust, adding more honey/ maple syrup + fresh tomato chunks, to taste.
6) Tip: Save sundried tomato soak water for today's dressing! (Raw "Thousand Island"!)

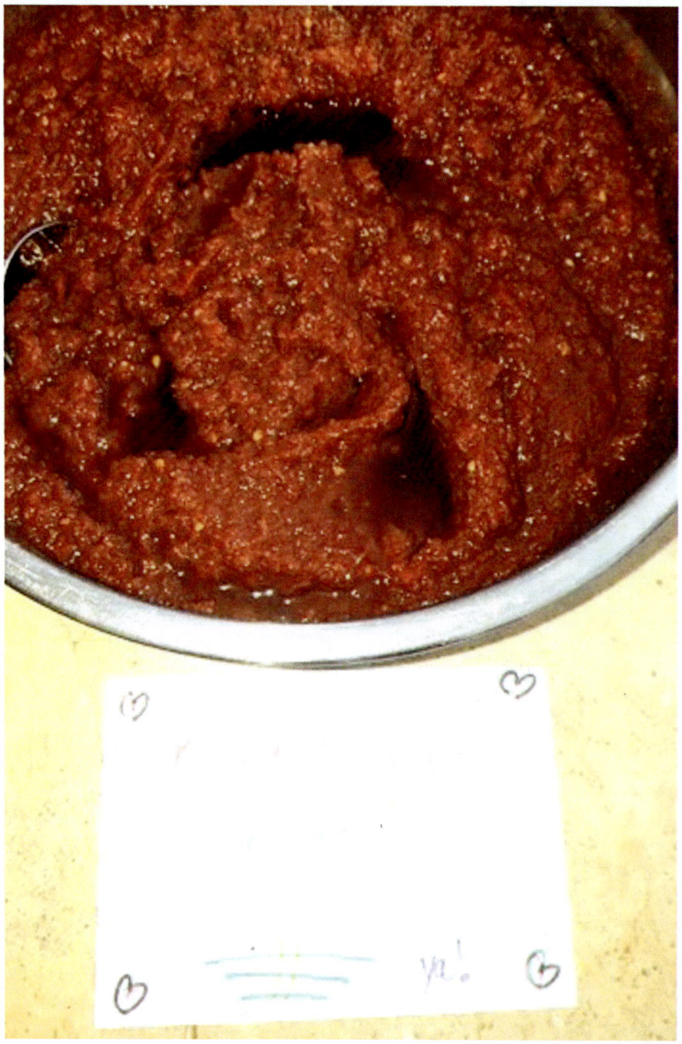

Roasted Rosemary Potatoes
Serves: 4
Time: 30 minutes

2 medium yellow potatoes
1 T olive oil
½ tsp sea salt
2 sprigs fresh rosemary

1) Cut potatoes into bite-size "chunks."
2) Add fresh rosemary (pulled from stem), olive oil + sea salt. Toss evenly, + roast @ 400 degrees till slightly golden brown. (You can add a splash of water to the bottom of the pan to "Steam/ Roast" for more plump potatoes, if desired. ;))

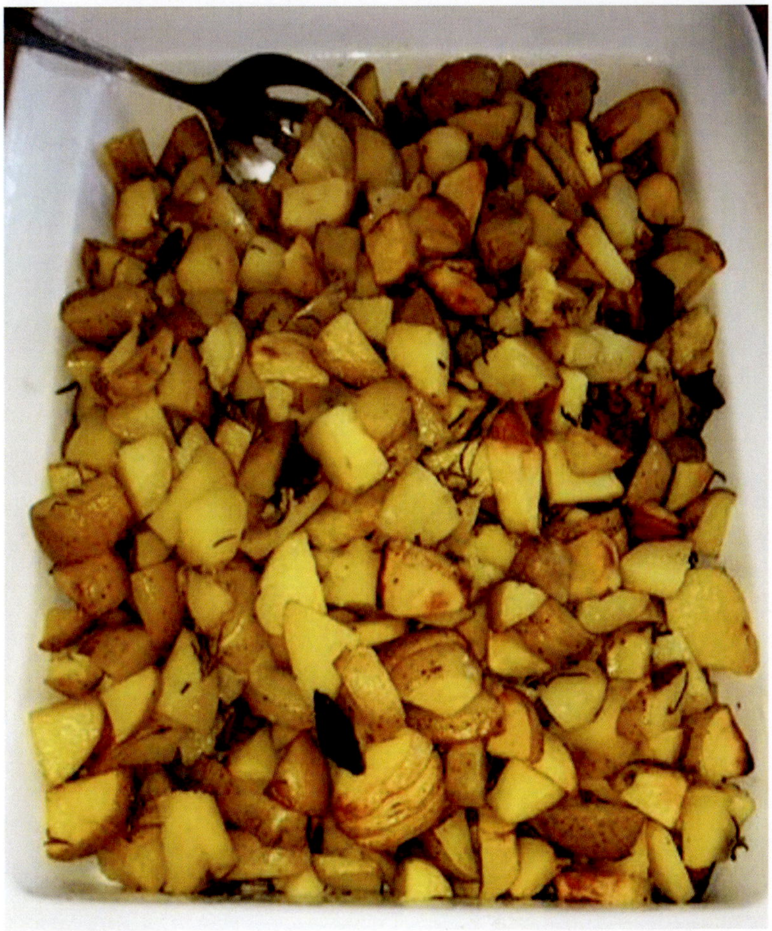

♥Green Salad

Serves: 4
Time: 15 minutes

1 head green/ red leaf lettuce, washed + broken into bite-size pieces
½ cucumber, thinly sliced into rounds
½ container Sunflower Sprouts

1) Arrange lettuce in a circular salad bowl.
2) Decorate with cucumber slices + sunflower sprouts in a mandala around the edges of the bowl.
3) Enjoy with Raw "Thousand Island" dressing! Simple + Easy!

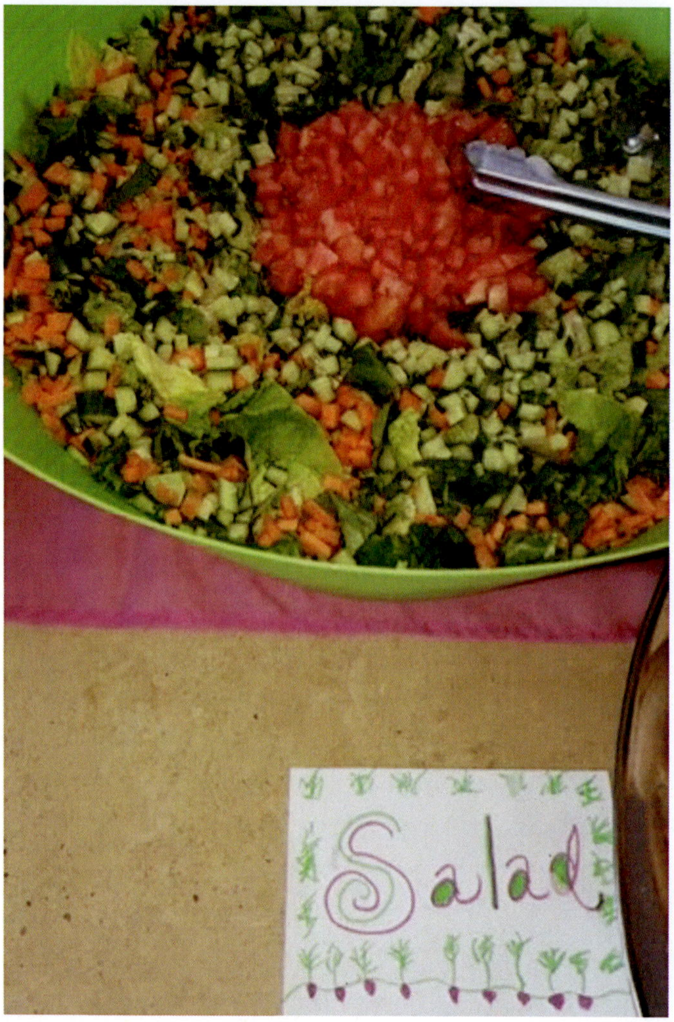

♥ΔRaw "Thousand Island" Dressing

Serves: 10
Time: 15 minutes (requires overnight soaking of cashews + sundried tomatoes)

1 c raw cashews, soaked
½ c sundried tomatoes, soaked
¼ c filtered water/ or sundried tomato soak water
4 T fresh-squeezed lemon juice
3 dates, pitted
1 tsp sea salt
1 tsp onion powder
½ tsp garlic powder
2 T apple cider vinegar
¼ c olive oil
1 Bubbies dill pickle

1) Soak cashews overnight, drain + rinse.
2) Blend all ingredients together (including pickle!). Yum Yum Yum!!! Enjoy!!
3) Tip: Dressing lasts 3-4 days in fridge. So, enjoy!

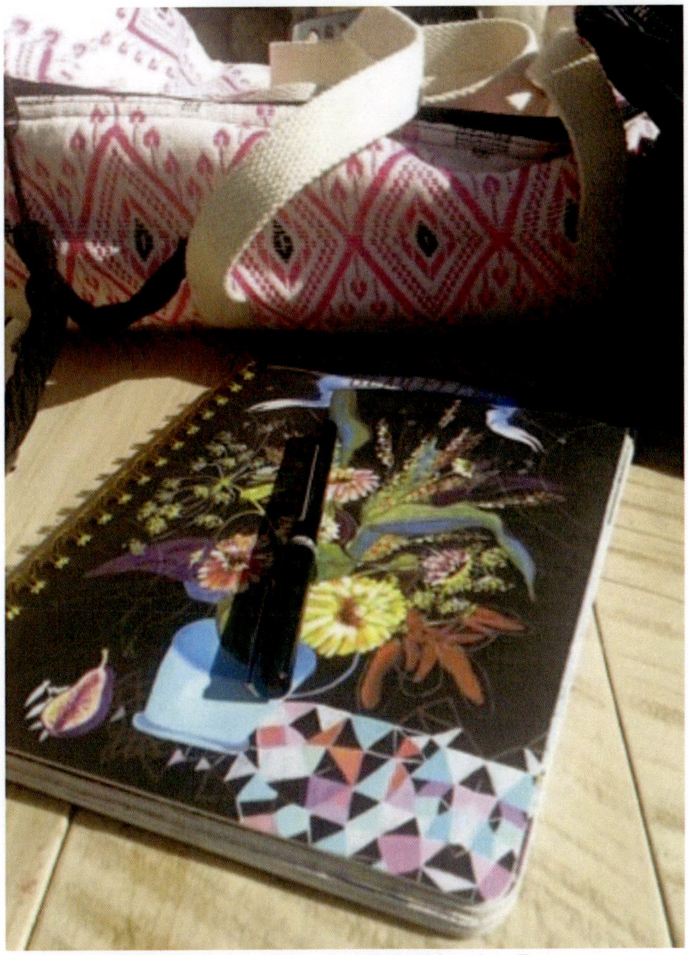

journaling before artist creation time/ the Morning Pages ♥

Tamale Night

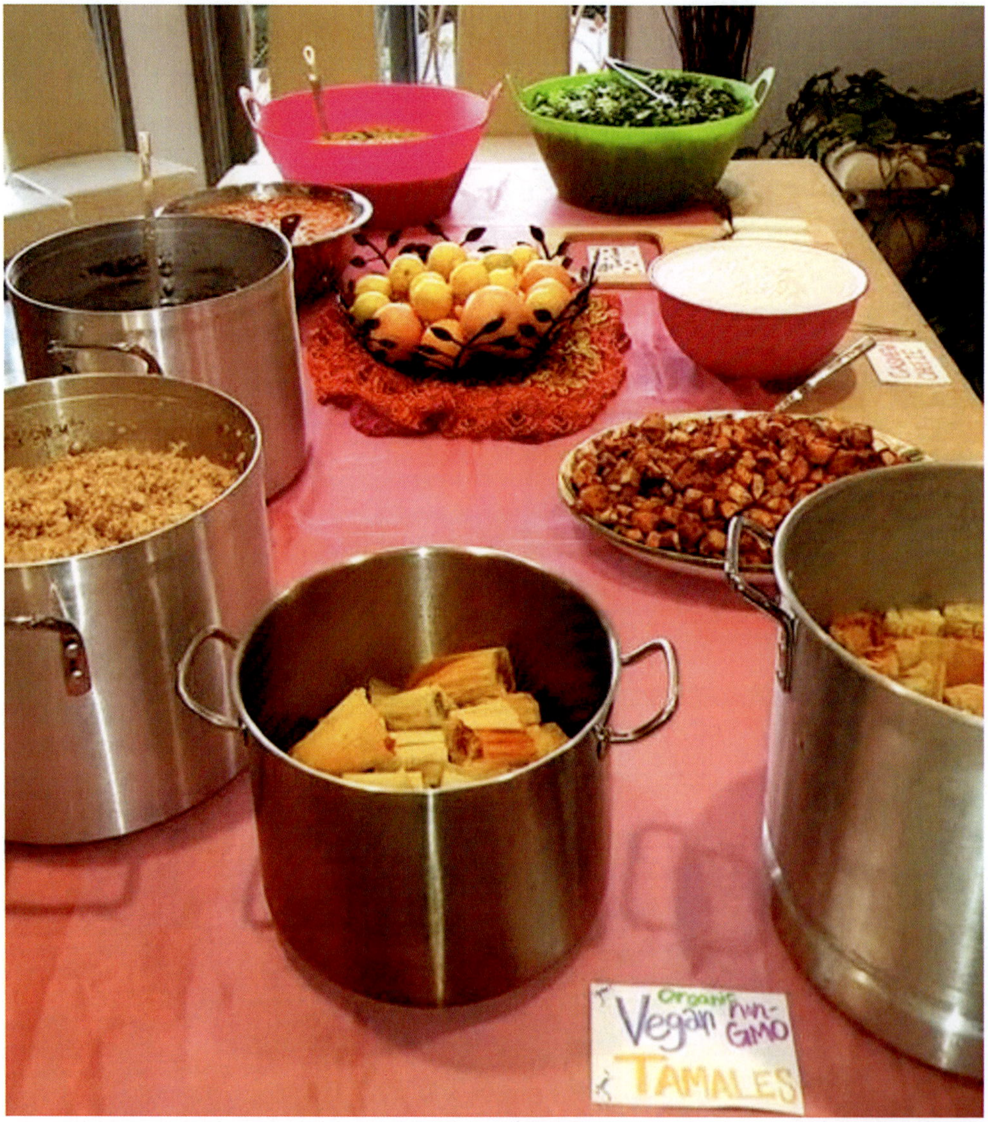

ΔCoconut Brown Rice

Serves: 6
Time: 45 minutes – 1 hour (requires overnight soaking of brown rice)

1 c Brown Rice, dry
1/3 c shredded coconut
1/3 tsp sea salt
1 T coconut oil
1/8 tsp cinnamon
1 pinch cayenne
2 ½ c water

1) Soak rice overnight, rinse + drain.
2) Cook 2 parts water/ 1 part soaked rice, on high. Add a lil' sea salt. Bring to a boil, turn down to low until cooked.
3) When rice is cooked, stir in all other ingredients, mix well, + serve! Yum!

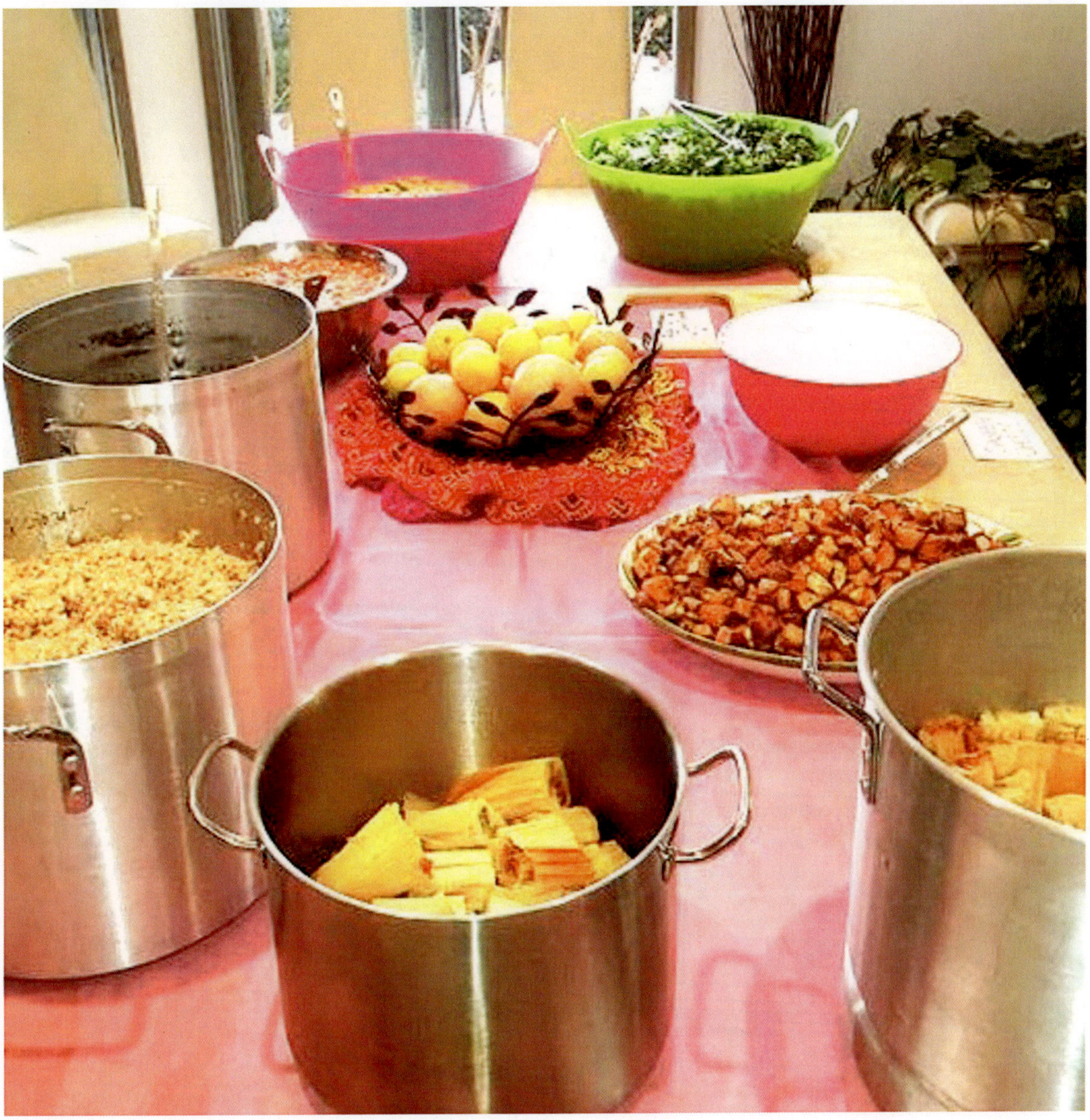

∆Black Beans

Serves: 8
Time: 1 hour (requires overnight soaking of beans)

2 c dry black beans (5 cups cooked)
1 tsp sea salt
2 cloves garlic
½ medium yellow onion, finely chopped
1 tomato
1 tsp cumin powder

1) Soak black beans overnight, drain + rinse.
2) Cook w/ filtered water about 4 inches above beans, with a pinch of sea salt, onions + pressed/ minced garlic!
3) Bring to a boil (on high), then reduce heat, add tomatoes, cumin powder + continue to cook until beans are soft. Optional: Add a splash of olive oil for flavor!
4) Enjoy!!

♥Salsa

Serves: 8
Time: 20 minutes

4 cups Tomato, cut into small "chunks"
1 Mango, cut into "chunks"
1 small Onion, finely chopped (can be Purple, Yellow, White, your choice!)
3 T fresh-squeezed lemon/ lime juice
1 tsp sea salt
1/5 bunch Cilantro, finely chopped
¼ hot pepper, minced
1 clove garlic, pressed/ minced

1) Chop tomatoes + mango into "chunks."
2) Chop onion + cilantro finely. Mince garlic + hot pepper.
3) Place all items in a mixing bowl. Stir in everything else + enjoy!

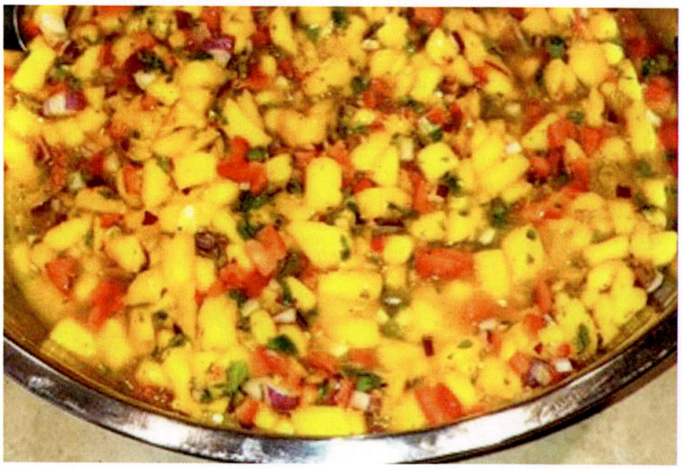

♥Guacamole
Serves: 10
Time: 20 minutes

4 Haas Avocados, cut into "chunks"
3 T fresh-squeezed lemon/ lime juice
1 small Onion, finely chopped (can be Purple, Yellow, White, your choice!)
1 T sea salt
1 medium Tomato, cut into small "chunks"
1/5 bunch cilantro, finely chopped
1 hot pepper, minced
1 clove garlic, pressed/ minced

1) Cut avocados + tomato into "chunks."
2) Chop onion, cilantro, hot peppers + garlic finely. (Food processor works great for garlic ;))
3) Place everything into a mixing bowl. Add all other ingredients, mix + enjoy.
4) If not eating right away, cover with lid + place in fridge so avocado stays fresh + green!

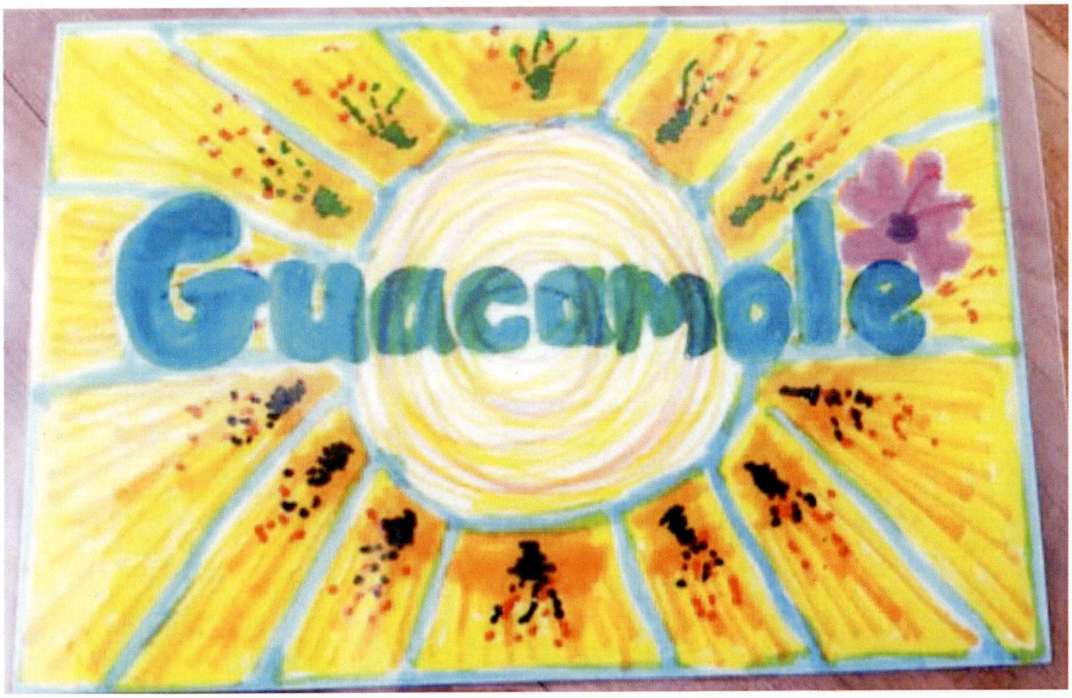

♥∆Raw Vegan Cashew Cheese
Serves: 8
Time: 15 minutes (requires overnight soaking of cashews)

3 c soaked raw cashews
1 c filtered water
¼ c fresh-squeezed lemon juice
1 t sea salt

1) Soak raw cashews overnight, drain + rinse.
2) Blend all ingredients together in Vitamix/ blender.
3) Serve + enjoy! Yum!

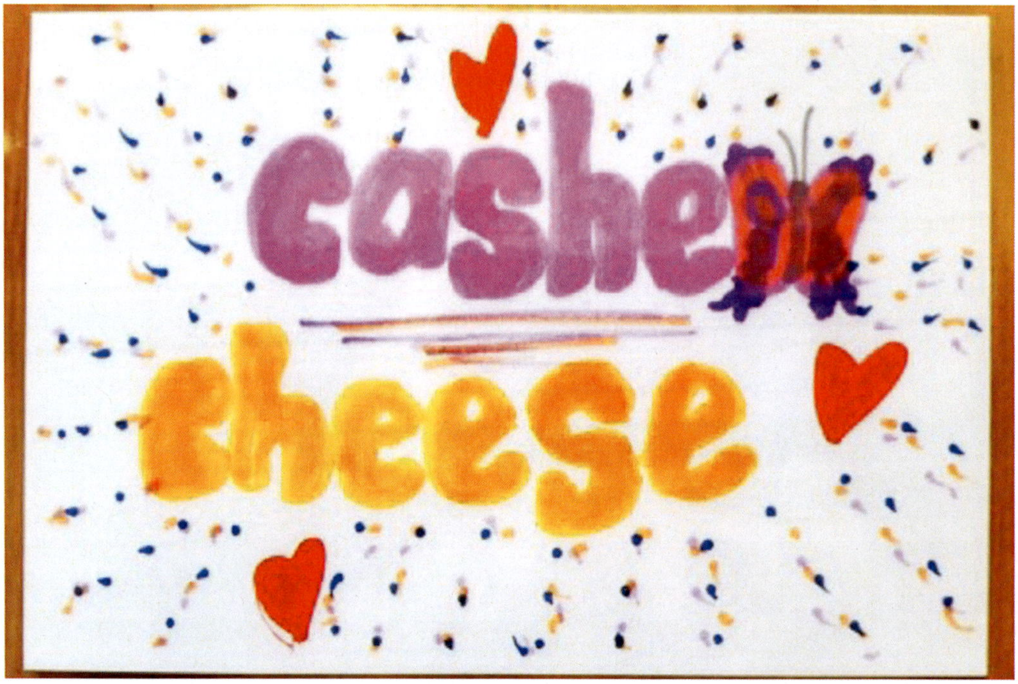

Other Meal Add-Ons

Serves: 4
Time: 15 minutes (plus Tamale ordering + pickup lol ;))

1 head Romaine lettuce, shredded
4 Vegan Organic Tamales (I purchase mine from Mother's Market + Kitchen in Costa Mesa/ Orange County!)

1) Shred the lettuce! (Wash + chop thin!)
2) Steam Tamales to heat, in a tamale steamer! Placing a couple of inches' water underneath the steamer, + lining up tamales vertically, open-side up. Steam for 15 minutes. Yum Yum!!

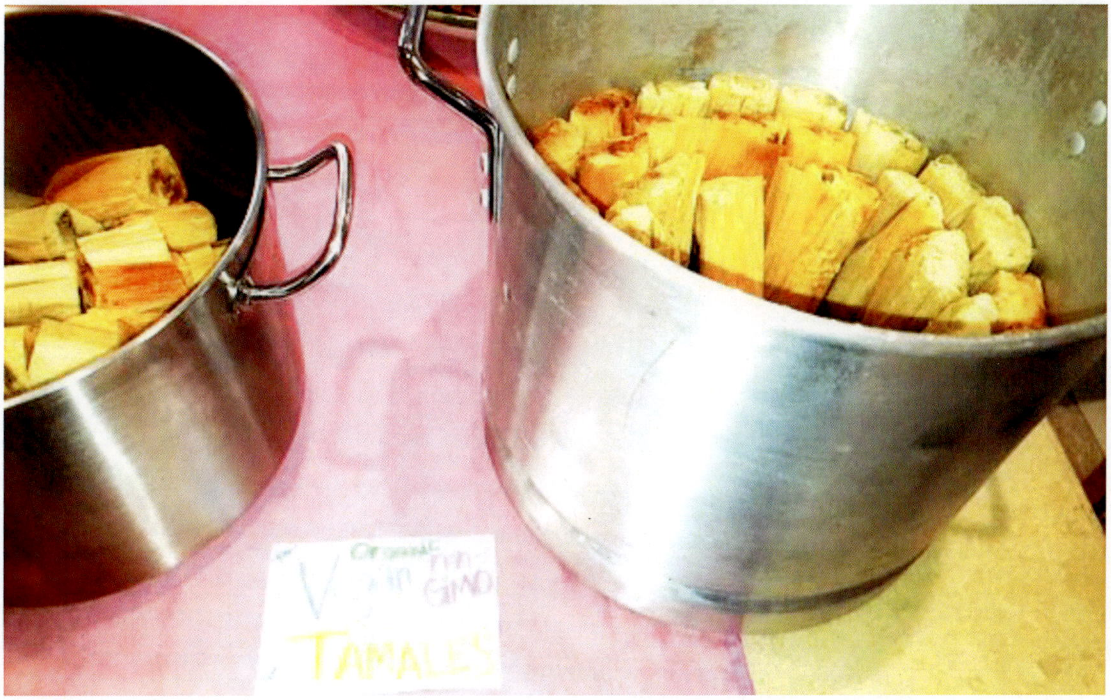

Kitchari Meal

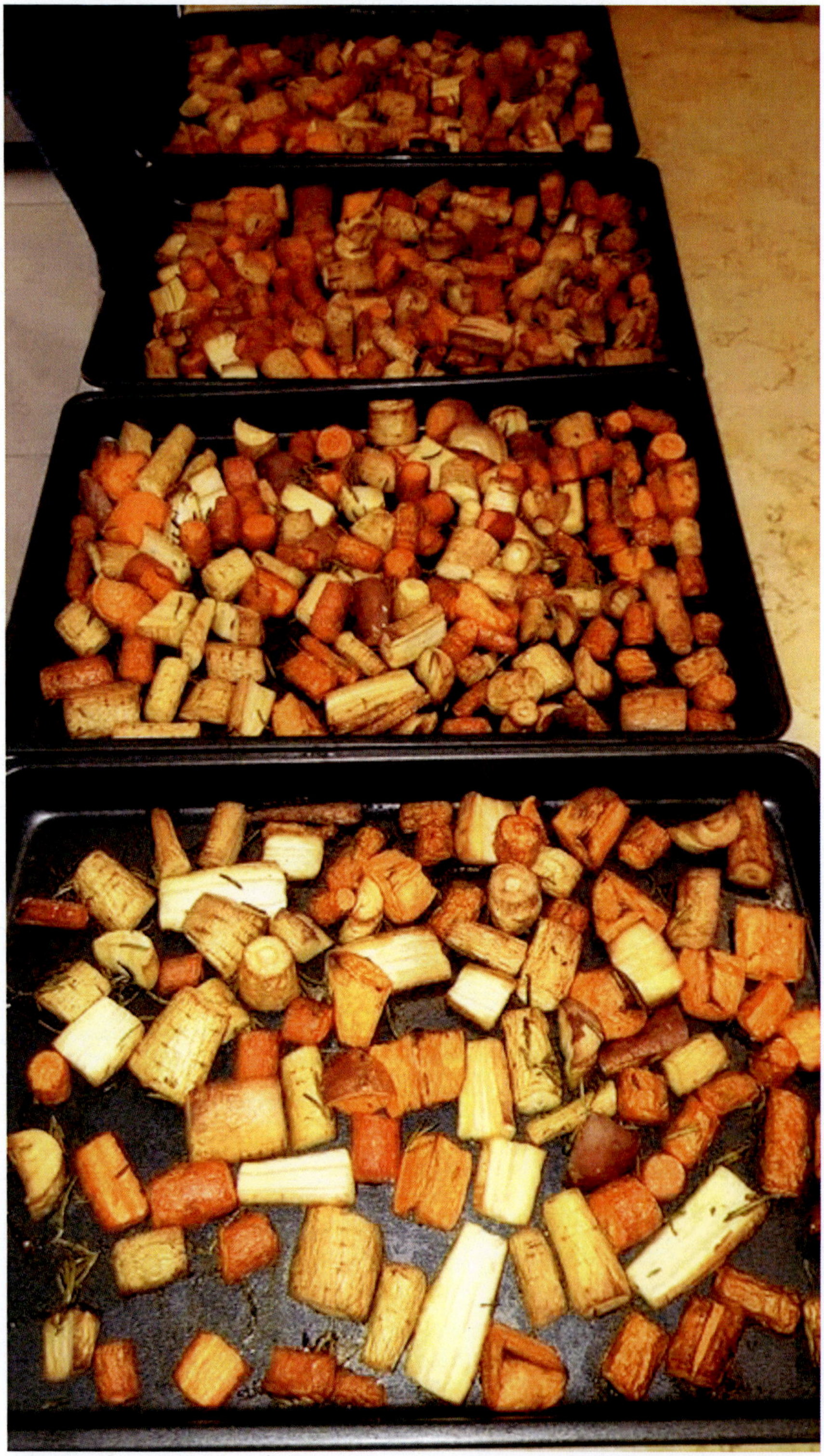

ΔSummer Squash Kitchari

Serves: 10
Time: 45 minutes – 1 hour (requires overnight soaking of rice + mung beans)

Some Kitchari recipes call for white rice, as it is more quickly assimilated into the body. However, I prefer brown rice, as it is the "original" rice, before the fiber has been stripped. You can adjust to your fancy, changing the spices too, as you desire.

1 c brown rice, dry
2 c mung dahl, dry
6 c filtered water
2 tsp cumin powder
2 tsp turmeric powder
2 tsp whole fennel seeds
2 tsp sea salt
1 tsp cinnamon
2 tsp fresh ginger, minced
1 zucchini/ summer squash, diced/ chopped
1 T coconut oil
1 tsp cardamom
1 tsp coriander
¼ yellow onion, chopped finely

1) Soak Rice + Mung Bean overnight, drain + rinse.
2) Begin cooking rice + mung beans w/ ginger + onion, + sea salt. (Optional to sauté fresh ginger + onion first in coconut oil + then add to the pot. ;))
3) Cook on high heat + bring to a boil. When boiling, turn heat to low + add vegetables + spices.
4) Cook until well-melded + yummy, stirring in coconut oil at the end. ;)
5) Optional: In wintertime, substitute butternut/ winter squash for summer squash! Add other seasonal vegetables such as kale, etc.

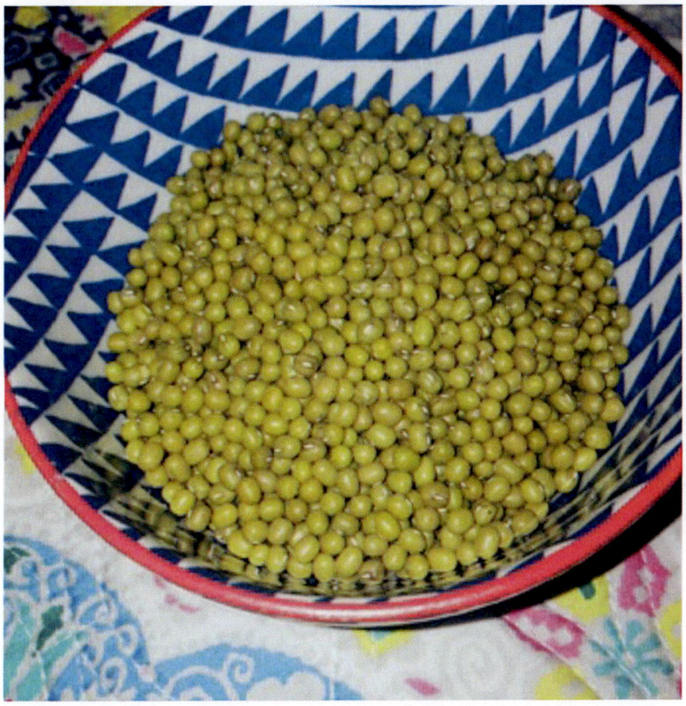

Roasted Sweet Potato, Parsnip + Carrot
Serves: 10
Time: 50 minutes

3 medium sweet potatoes, cut into “chunks”
1 lb carrots (about 10), cut into “chunks”
5 medium parsnips, cut into “chunks”
3 T coconut oil
1 tsp cinnamon
½ tsp sea salt

1) Cut roots into chunks. Place into a mixing bowl.
2) Toss w/ coconut oil, cinnamon, sea salt.
3) Bake @ 350-400 degrees on a coconut-oiled baking ban/ or glass dish.
4) When kitchen starts smelling great, check w/ fork to see if they are done!
5) Enjoy! You can be sweet, without desserts! ;) Try it!

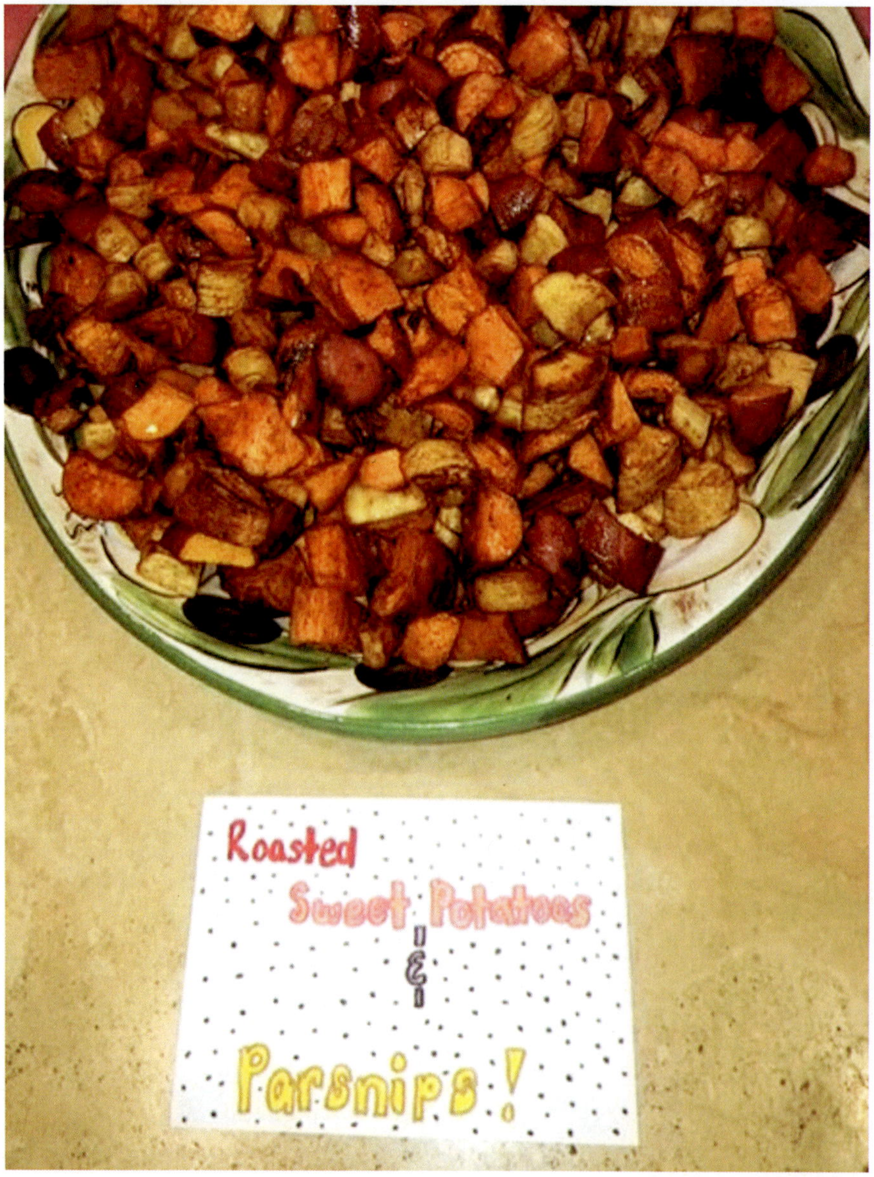

♥Kale Salad Classic

Serves: 3
Time: 15 minutes

This recipe is one my claims to fame, appearing in a front-page article in the Atlanta Journal-Constitution over seven years ago! It is one of the easiest, simplest recipes to make, while still being hearty + filling. I like to wrap this in a raw nori sheet + take it on the go!

1 bunch Kale, chopped into bite-size pieces
½ Avocado, cut into "chunks"
1 T fresh-squeezed lemon juice
1 T olive oil
½ tsp sea salt
1 clove garlic, minced/ pressed

1) Break/ chop kale lovingly into bite-size bits.
2) Massage ingredients with hands in a big bowl until wilted + marinated. (Personally, I like to wait + massage everything except avocado, then add that last, to maintain "chunk" texture. ;))
3) Remember your healing reiki hands.

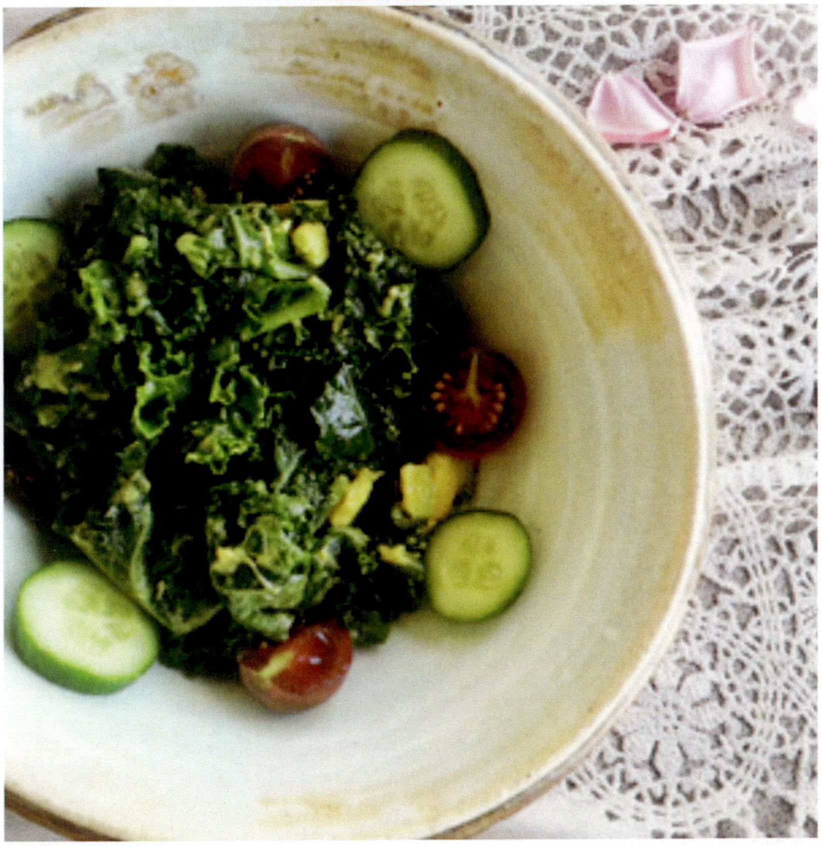

♥ΔRaw Vegan Strawberry Cake – inspired by Matthew Rogers' + Tiziana Alipo Tamborra's Strawberry Shortcake, Sweet Gratitude (get the book!)
Serves: 20
Time: a really long-ass time ;) 1 ½ hours (45 minutes to make, 1 hour to chill, requires soaking cashews overnight)

Cake:
2 lbs dates, pitted
¾ c coconut oil, melted
3 T vanilla extract
1 tsp sea salt
8 c almond flour (can buy raw almond flour, or use almond pulp from making raw almond mylk ;))
3 c strawberries

Icing:
2 c cashews, dry, soaked overnight
2 c coconut milk (to make "raw" coconut milk, blend young coconut water + meat)
½ c raw local honey
1 T fresh-squeezed lemon juice
1 T vanilla extract
1 pinch sea salt
2 T sunflower lecithin (this is a soy-free vegan thickener)
1 c coconut oil, melted

For Cake:

1) Wash + de-stem strawberries. Pit dates carefully, including stem.
2) Food process dates, vanilla, sea salt, 2 c strawberries, coconut oil, a lil at a time to keep food processor turning (in batches).
3) Stir in almond flour + 1 c sliced strawberries for the cake part.
4) Refrigerate cake batter for 30 minutes.

For Icing:

1) Soak cashews overnight, drain + rinse.
2) Blend all ingredients in Vitamix/ blender, except lecithin + coconut oil.
3) When smooth, add sunflower lecithin + coconut oil last to thicken. Refrigerate to chill/ set.
4) Keep icing in the fridge for 30 minutes – 1 hour to "set."

To Assemble Cake:

1) Divide cake batter into half, for 2 cake layers, Roll bottom cake batter into a ball + pat flat with hands onto cake plate. Meanwhile, get the 2nd layer ready by flattening/ shaping onto a glass pie pan or plate. You can use plastic wrap underneath so it comes off easily. ;) Add icing to bottom cake layer, then flip 2nd cake layer on top of iced 1st layer.
2) Ice cake, adding strawberries, sliced or whole, to decorate on top. Light candles + sing "Happy Birthday!" ;) Yay! You did it!!

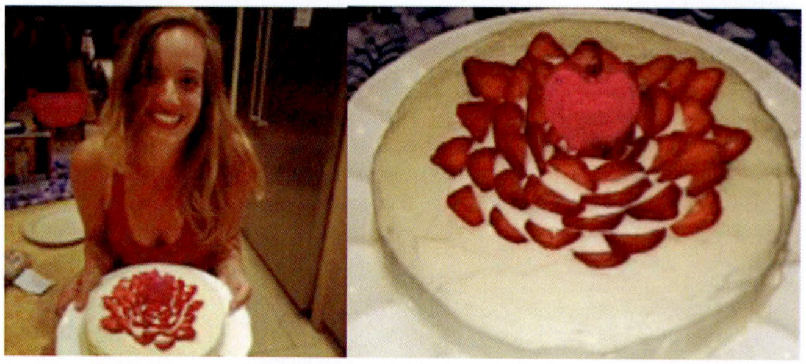

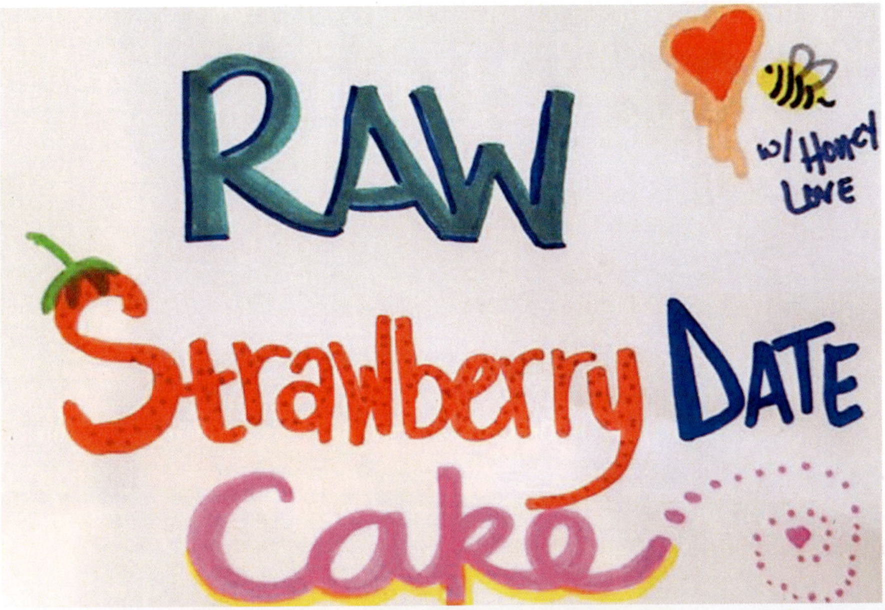
RAW
w/ Honey
Love
Strawberry DATE
Cake

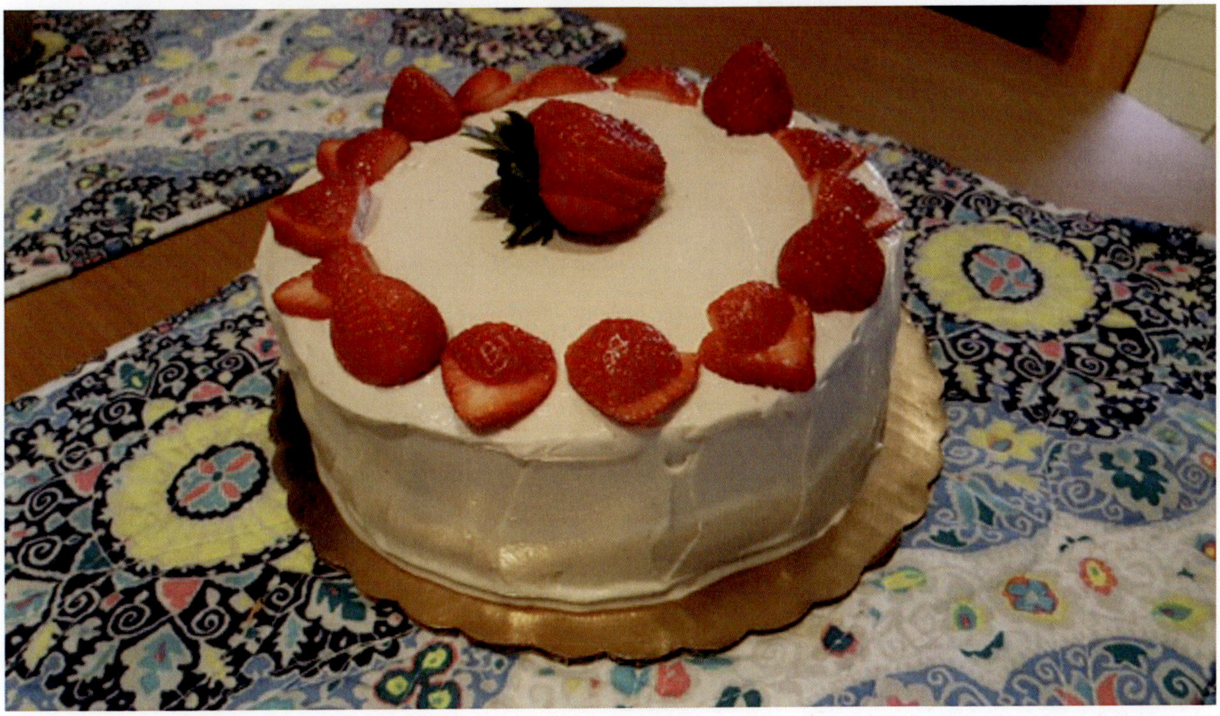

Soul Food Night

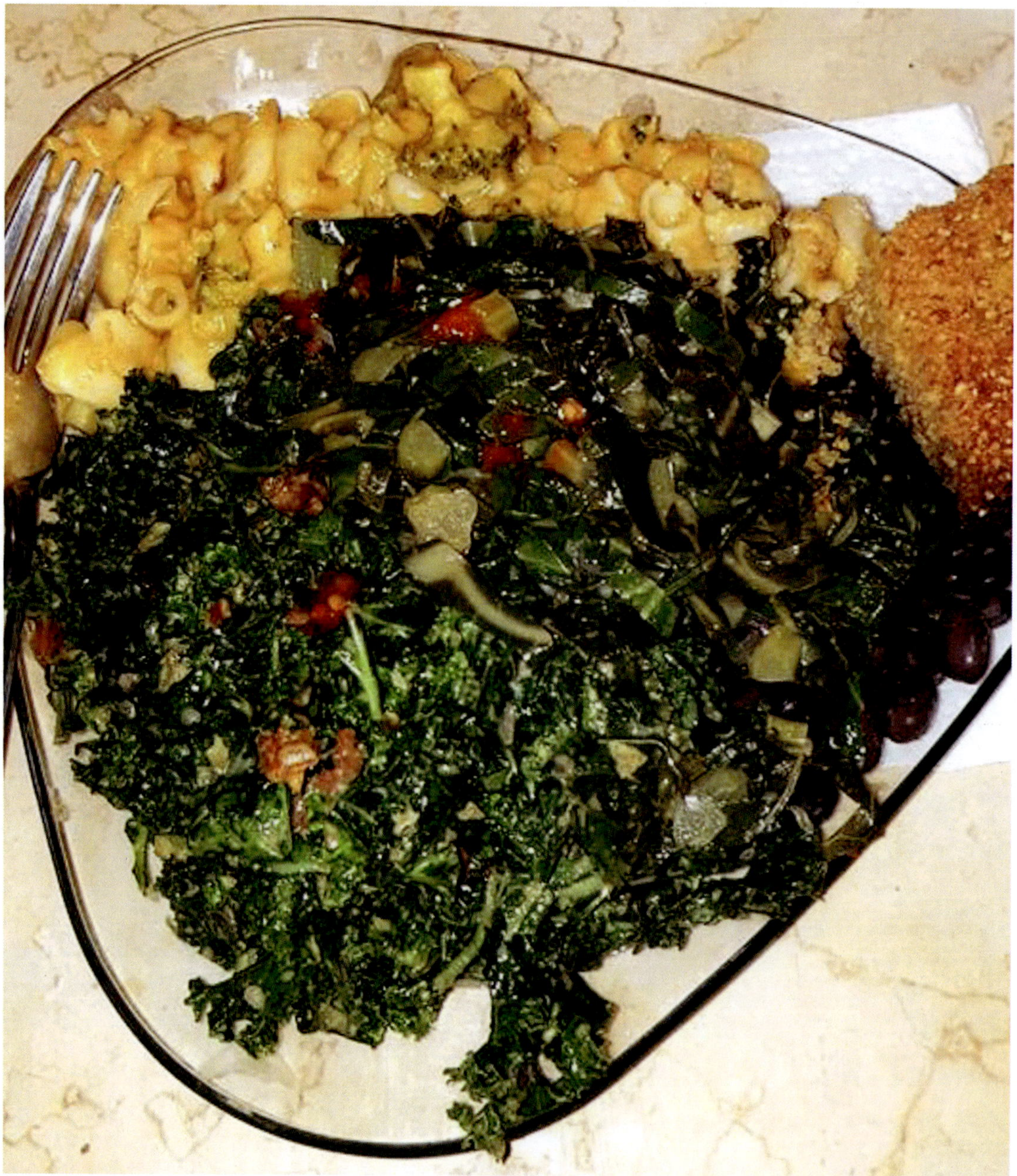

ΔYellow Lentil Soul Patties

Serves: 4
Time: 40 minutes (requires overnight soaking of lentils)

2 c yellow lentils, soaked
2 carrots, cut into "chunks"
¼ red bell pepper, cut into "chunks"
1/8 onion
¼ tsp sea salt
1/8 tsp black or cayenne pepper
1/8 bunch parsley
2 T coconut oil

1) Food process onion + fresh parsley till fine, then add carrots + red bell peppers. When this is processed, add soaked yellow lentils, salt + pepper. Add a pinch of filtered water if needed, to turn.
2) Pour/ rubber scrape Yellow Lentil Soul Patty "batter" into a mixing bowl.
3) Heat a frying pan w/ Coconut Oil. Make Soul Patty "balls" with your hands, flatten, + then place carefully in the frying pan. Fry till golden brown, flipping to bless both sides! Mmm… enjoy!

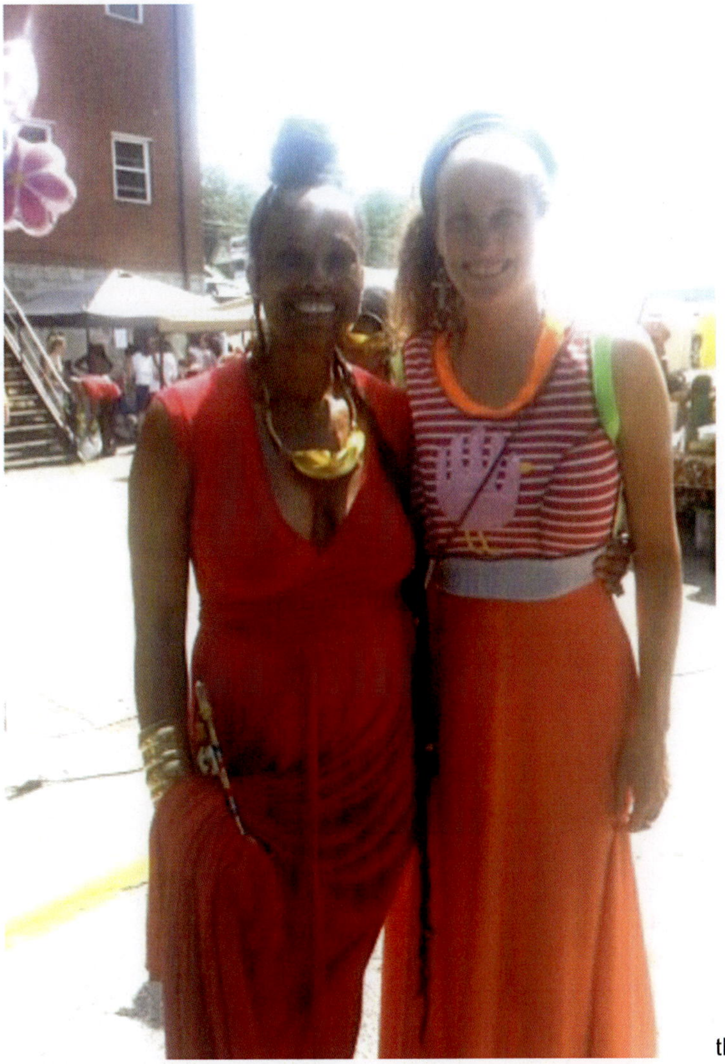

the beautiful Tassili @ Tassili's Raw Reality

Vegan Gluten-Free (Soy-Free Everything-Free Yet Amazing) Mac + Cheese - inspired by Vegan Richa, Vegan Black Pepper Mac + Cheese w/ Potato Carrot Cheese Sauce, VeganRicha.com!!
Serves: 3
Time: 45 minutes

2 ½ cups filtered water
1 medium potato
1/3 c carrots
4 cloves garlic
1/8 fresh onion
½ green chili
½ medium tomato, cut in "chunks"
½ tsp prepared wet mustard (I love Eden Organics brand!)
2 tsp Bragg's liquid aminos
4 T nutritional yeast
2 tsp fresh-squeezed lemon juice
2 T olive oil
1/3 tsp paprika
¾ tsp sea salt
¾ tsp black pepper
8 oz elbow pasta (I love Pastariso brand gluten-free Brown Rice Pasta Elbows)
1 c fresh broccoli, chopped into bite-size pieces

1) Boil potatoes + carrots till soft. Drain water.
2) Blend everything except pasta + broccoli! (This becomes your Sauce! ;)) Do in batches if you're making multiples of this recipe (you may want to, because it is SOOOO good! One of my favorites in this book! ;))
3) Boil water for pasta. Cook pasta according to directions on package.
4) When there is a minute left of pasta cooking, throw in chopped broccoli (bite-sized pieces) + steam in pasta water (Yes, *with* the pasta! ;))
5) When finished, drain pasta + broccoli.
6) Stir in cheese sauce + Serve! (OMG! I LOOOVE this recipe!!! YUM YUM (healthy) Comfort Food!) Thank You Vegan Richa for being so Amazing! I recommend you buy her recipe book too! ;))

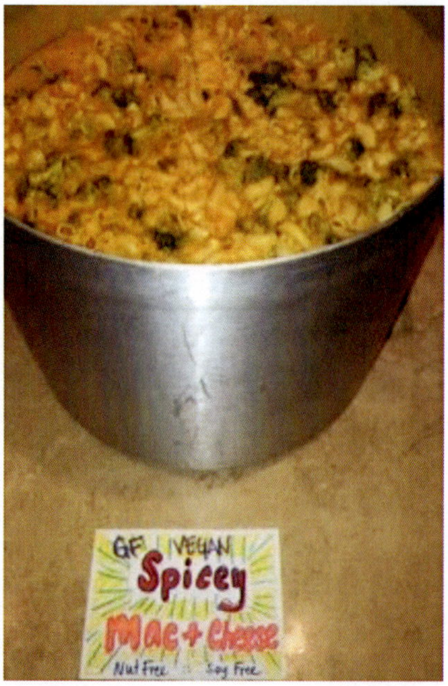

Southern Collard Greens
Serves: 3
Time: 15 minutes (yes, that's it!!)

1 bunch collard greens
1 T Bragg's liquid aminos
¼ yellow onion, sliced thin
2 cloves garlic, optional
1 T coconut oil
splash hot sauce

1) Sauté finely chopped onion (+ optional garlic) in coconut oil till translucent.
2) Cut collards into ribbons. (It's okay, for cooked greens, to include the stem.)
3) Add greens to pan.
4) Add Bragg's + splash of hot sauce.
5) When greens turn bright green (not brown/ overcooked), Serve + Enjoy!!

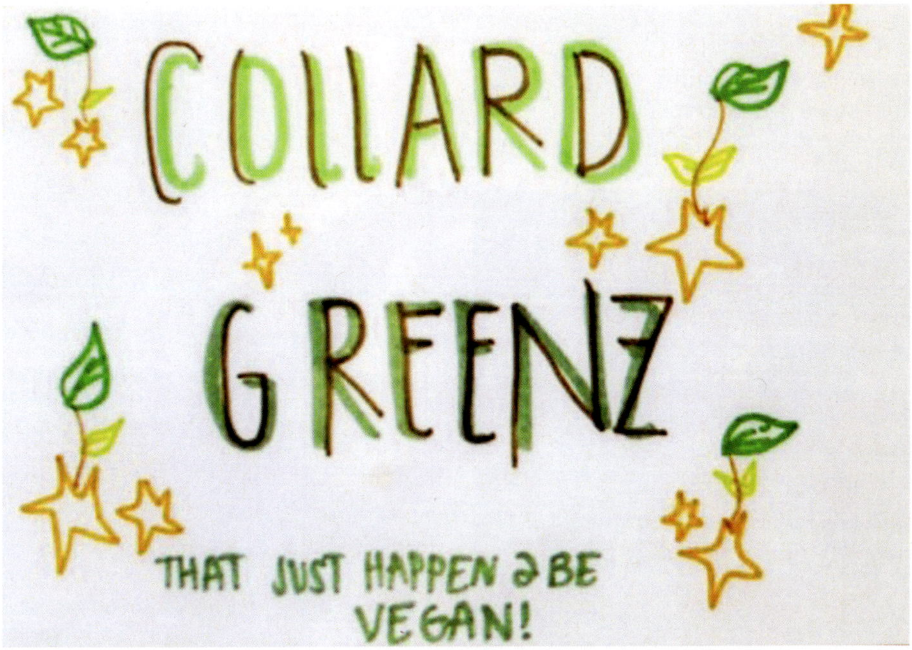

♥∆Spicy Kale

Serves: 4
Time: 15 minutes (requires overnight soaking of sundried tomatoes)

This recipe is inspired by mouth-watering memories of Tassili's Raw Reality restaurant in Atlanta! (I tried to channel the kale, Tassili!) Visit Tassili's whenever you're in town! ;)

1 bunch curly green kale, washed, de-stemmed, + cut into bite-sized pieces
½ c soaked sundried tomatoes, sliced thin
¼ red onion, sliced thin
1 clove garlic, pressed/ minced
¼ tsp cayenne pepper
1/5 c nutritional yeast
1 T fresh-squeezed lemon juice
½ t sea salt
1 T olive oil

1) Soak sundried tomatoes overnight in water (covered just enough to top tomatoes).
2) Wash + cut kale (de-stemmed) into bite-sized pieces. (You can save the stems for juicing!) Put kale in large mixing bowl.
3) Cut soaked sundried tomatoes into strips + add to kale.
4) Cut red onion into thin strips + add to mix.
5) Add all other ingredients + massage, adjusting till yummy!

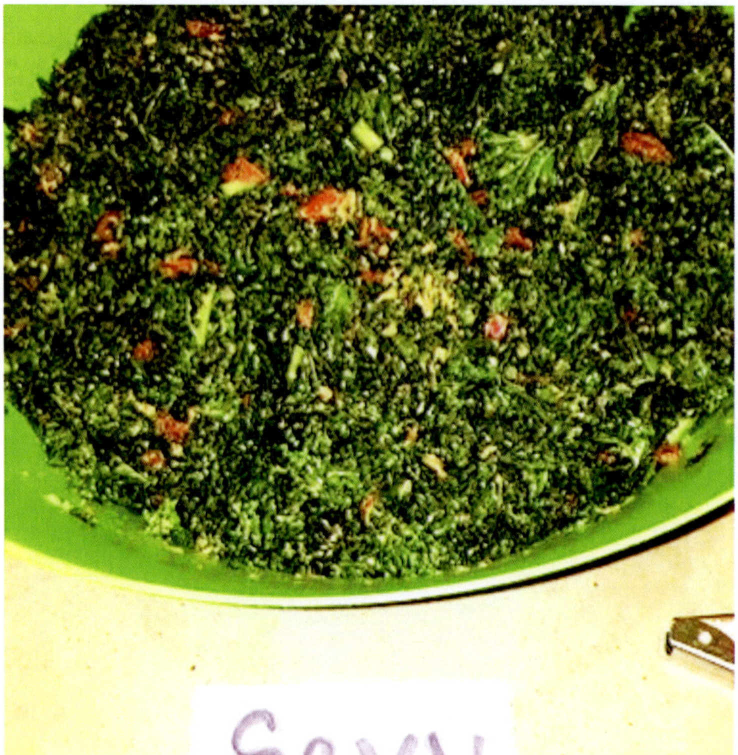

Mashed Sweet Potatoes

Serves: 4
Time: 40 minutes (mostly baking/ cooking time, about 10 minutes' prep! ;))

1 large sweet potato
1 T Grade B maple syrup
¼ tsp cinnamon
1 pinch sea salt
¼ c coconut milk/ or filtered water if blending!

1) Cut sweet potato into chunks + boil in water until soft (about 20-30 minutes). Or, you can also roast sweet potato, covered in coconut oil + sea salt, till soft, about 30 minutes.
2) In food processor, blend all ingredients together till yummy. OR, if roasted, a yummy alternative is to leave in chunks + drizzle with maple syrup + cinnamon, stirring till mixed! YUM!

Gluten-Free Cornbread

Serves: 16 (1 square sheet pan)
Time: 45 minutes (including baking time ;))

1 1/5 c coconut milk
2 c fine cornmeal
1 T apple cider vinegar
2 T baking powder
1 tsp sea salt
½ tsp baking soda
¼ c Grade B maple syrup
1 small bag frozen organic corn
2 T coconut oil
1/3-1/2 c organic applesauce

1) Mix all wet ingredients in a bowl.
2) Mix all dry ingredients in another separate bowl.
3) Mix wet + dry together.
4) Bake in a coconut oil-greased square pan @ 350 degrees for 20 minutes.
5) Check w/ fork + see if it's done! (If fork comes out clean, it's done! Thanks Mom for teaching me that! ;))
6) Cool, cut into squares, + serve! Yum Yum!! Pairs so well with everything else!

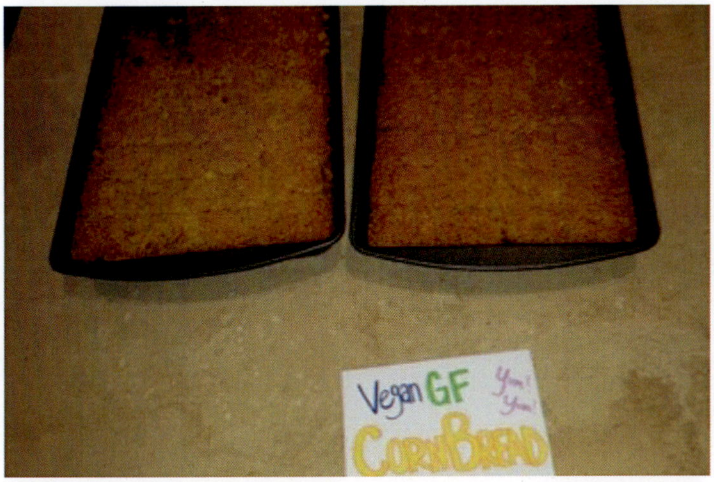

Breakfast/ Brunch

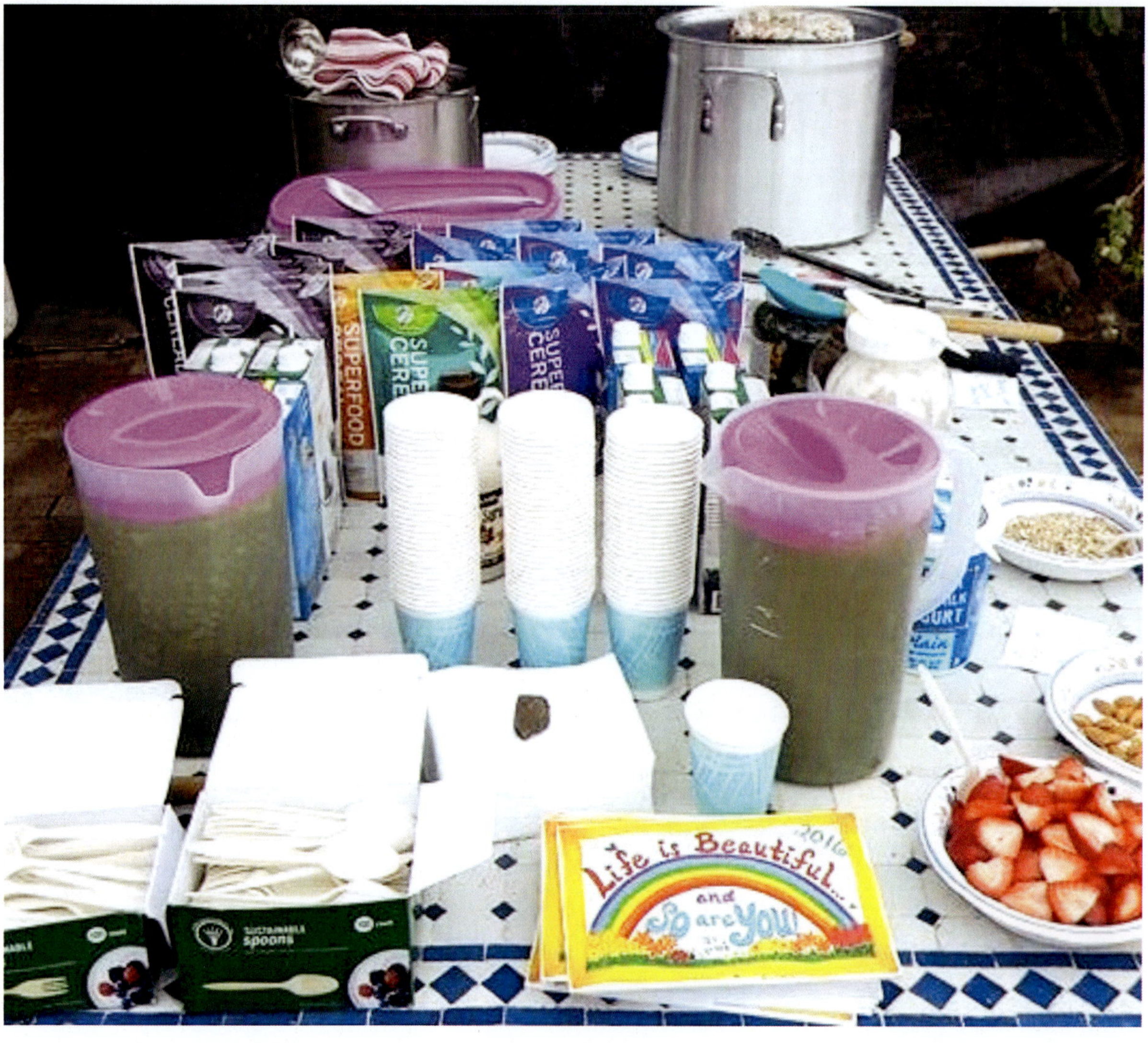

Beautiful Calendars by istandforlove.com ♥

♥Green Superfood Smoothie
Serves: 6
Time: 15 minutes

2 cups seasonal fruit (apples, peaches, oranges are great!)
1 small avocado, sliced, pitted + scooped
2 cups leafy greens, washed (kale or lettuce is great!)
2 T protein powder (I love Vega, Billy's Infinity Greens, Healthforce Nutritionals, Medicinal Foods Living Greens, + so much more!)
1 T green powder (see above! I also love Garden of Life!)
filtered water to 8 cup line (including other ingredients!)
2 T raw local honey

1) Pit + scoop avocado. Peel oranges/ cut/ or pit any fruit. Cut fruit into big chunks, wash lettuce.
2) Put all ingredients into Vitamix, then fill to 8 cup line with filtered water.
3) Blend until smooth + enjoy!! 1 minute does the trick (or less!)

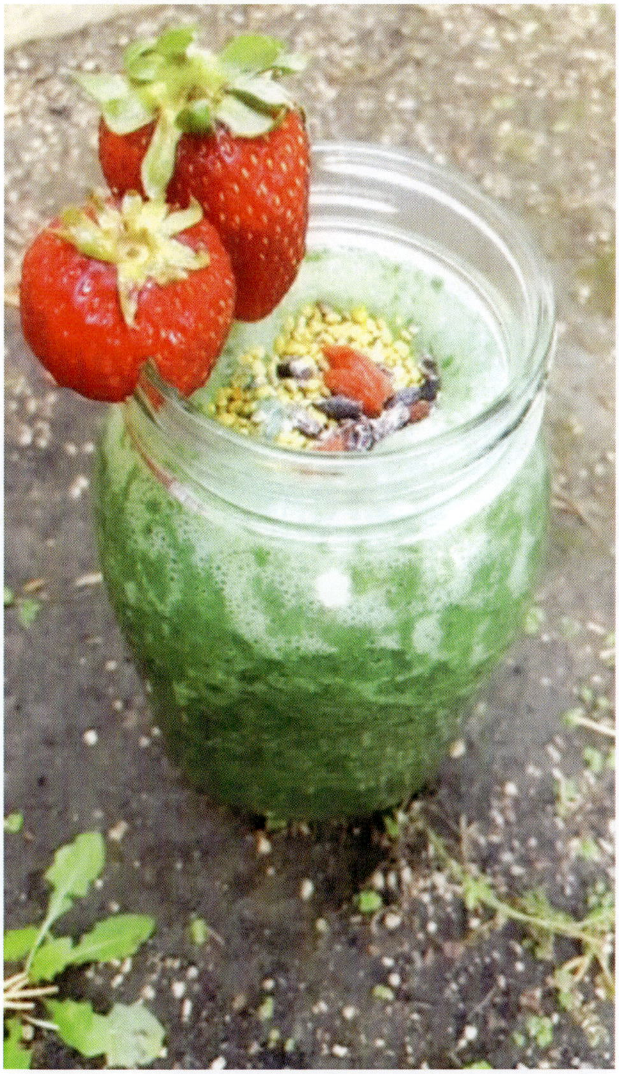

Warm Cardamom Raisin Quinoa Porridge
Serves: 4
Time: 25 minutes

1 c Quinoa, dry
2 c filtered water
1 tsp cinnamon
1 tsp cardamom
1/3 c raisins
pinch sea salt
½ tsp vanilla extract
1 ½ T Grade B maple syrup
2 T slivered almonds
1/3 can coconut milk (optional)

1) Cook quinoa along with dry raisins (to allow them to plump in the water).
2) Bring to a boil, then reduce heat to low. Then add spices, vanilla, sea salt, maple syrup. Adjust to your taste! Add coconut milk (optional).
3) Keep slivered almonds on the side, to top. Garnish + enjoy!! Yum, warm comfort food! Healthy breakfast! xoxoxo

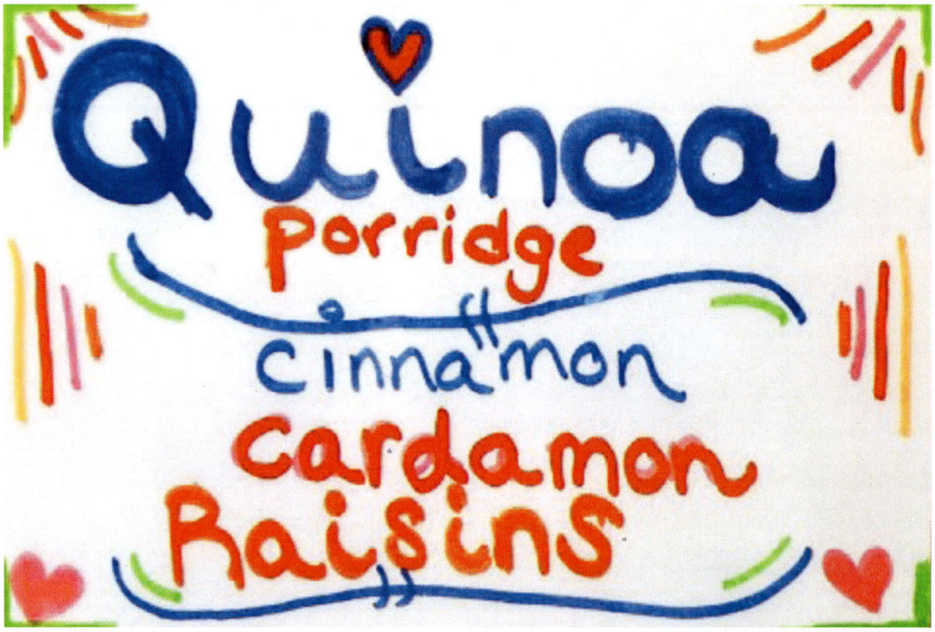

♥Living Intentions Sprouted Granola + Almond/ Coconut Milk

Serves: 5
Time: 5 min!

Living Intentions is an amazing brand I love! Plus, they happen to be dear friends of mine! And I love your whole crew too! Their sprouted raw granola makes a great addition to a retreat breakfast – for many guests, or within your own home. ;)

1 bag Living Intentions Sprouted Granola
1 carton Almond/ Coconut Milk

1) Serve + enjoy!! A little goes a long way! Especially when served with other items! ;) xo

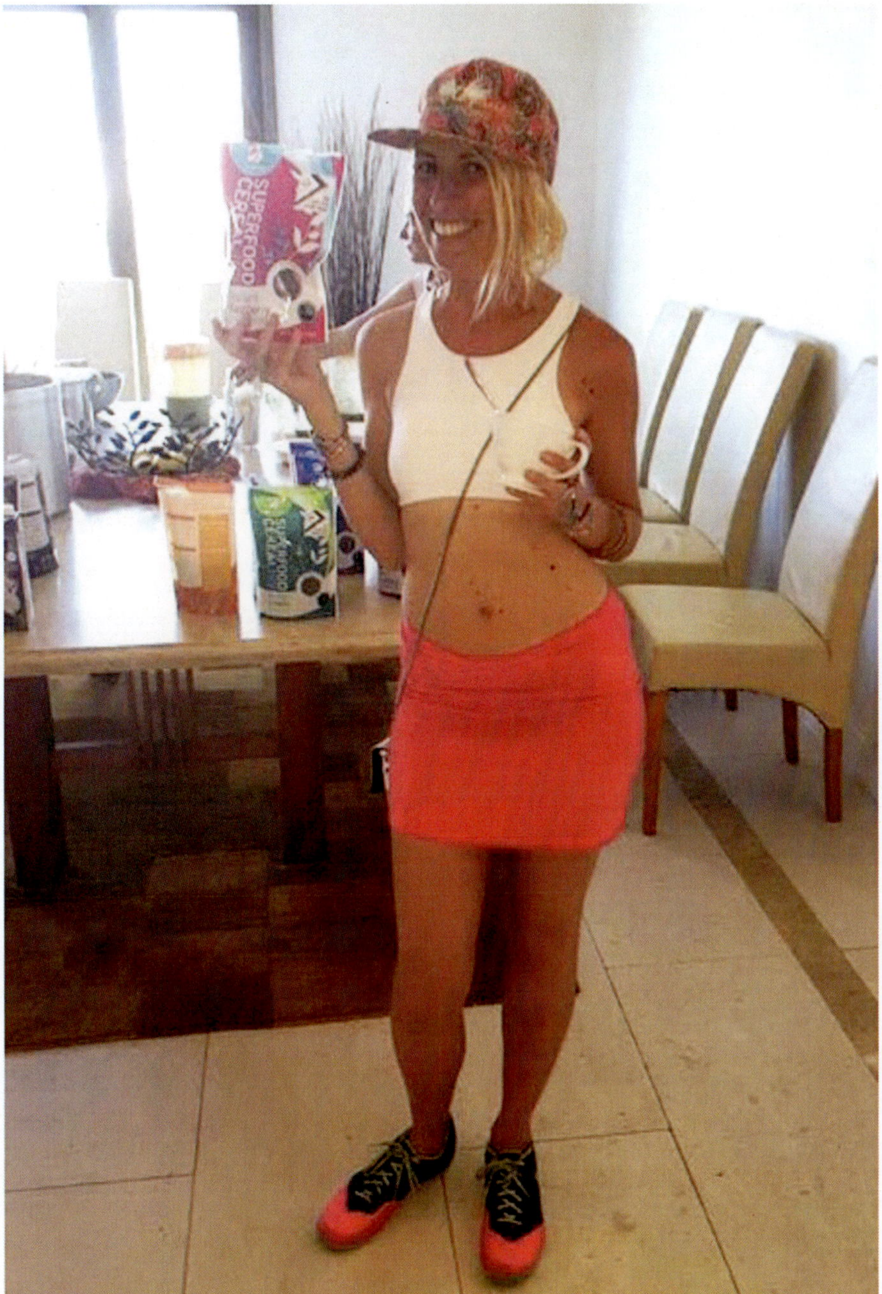

Sushi Lunch

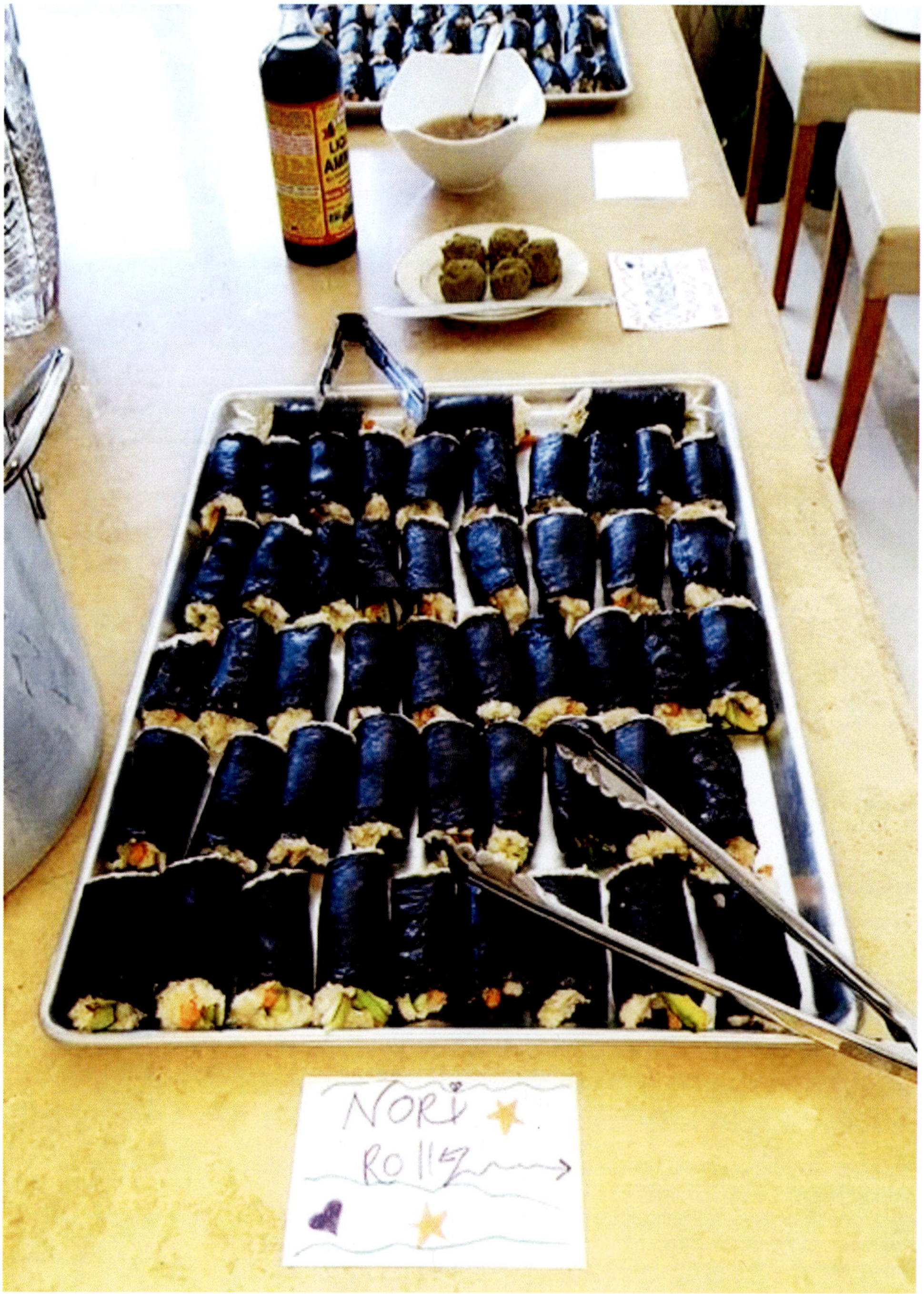

ΔSushi Rice

Serves: 6
Time: 1 hour (requires overnight soaking of rice, + also refrigeration time ;))

1 c Brown Rice
3 c filtered water
1 T toasted sesame oil
1 T rice vinegar
1 T raw local honey/ Grade B maple syrup
1/3 t + a pinch sea salt
3 T untoasted brown sesame seeds

1) Soak brown rice overnight. Drain + rinse.
2) Cook brown rice in filtered water, with a pinch of salt.
3) When rice is done, mix in toasted sesame oil, rice vinegar, sweetener, sesame seeds + 1/3 t sea salt. Refrigerate overnight. The next day, it will be ready for rolling sushi!

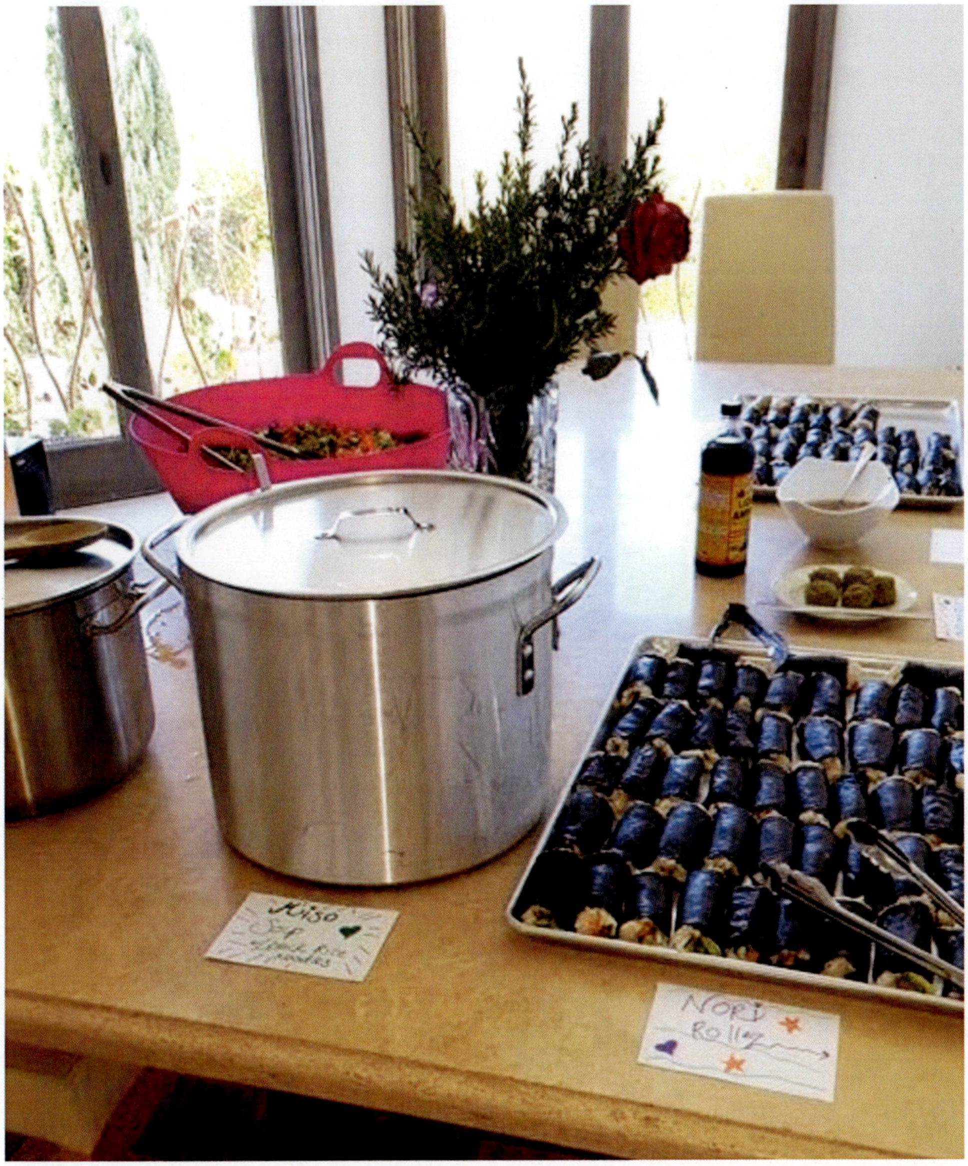

Sushi Ingredients + Rolling Sushi

Serves: 6
Time: 1 hour

6 Raw Untoasted Nori Wrappers (can be toasted, just my preference ;))
1 Avocado, sliced thin
1 cucumber, sliced into thin matchsticks
2 carrots, sliced into thin matchsticks
½ daikon radish, sliced into thin matchsticks
1 package sprouts (I love alfalfa or Sunflower, pick your fave! ;))
1 package Eden brand pickled ginger (all natural, no sugar ;))
1 package Eden brand dry Wasabi powder, mixed with filtered water as indicated on package (I've found that sometimes it requires more water to get to that balled-up, dry but slightly juicy consistency ;)
2/3 c Bragg's liquid aminos, for dipping!

1) Cut all vegetables as indicated, into matchsticks, slices.
2) Lay out nori wrapper, horizontally + smooth side down.
3) Smooth rice from the right to the left, all the way to the edges. Leave an inch of black at the bottom + 3-4 inches at the top.
4) Lay out all vegetables horizontally as indicated. Then roll sushi starting at the bottom, to the top. The first roll-over should cover all the vegetables. Roll up + pull tight. I always like to think of a beautiful whale, with tight smooth skin, when I roll sushi! ;)
5) Use ginger, wasabi, + Bragg's for dipping! Yum, yum! Enjoy!!

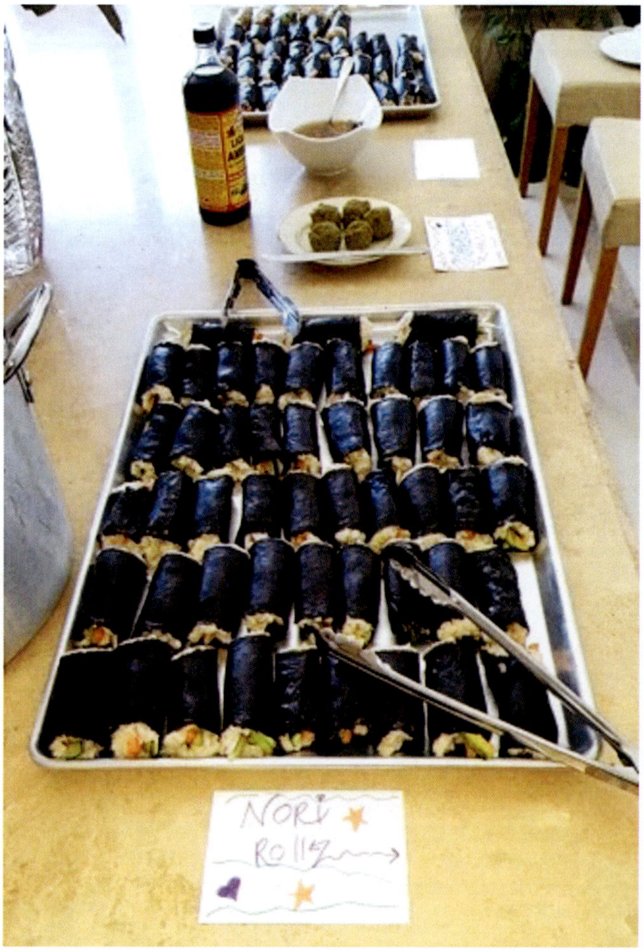

Chickpea Miso Soup w/ Bok Choi, Spinach, Black Rice Noodles, + Mushrooms
Serves: 6
Time: 45 minutes

1 head bok choi, washed + chopped in ribbons
¼ container chickpea miso (this is nice b/c it's soy-free! I love Miso Master brand ;))
½ bunch fresh spinach, washed + chopped if large leaves
1/3 bunch green onions, chopped finely
1 package black rice noodles (or use kelp noodles if you prefer ;)) (I love Lotus Foods Forbidden Rice Ramen!)
1 c mushrooms, washed + sliced
1 t fresh ginger, minced
1 clove garlic, pressed/ minced
1 T ume plum vinegar (This is a great chef's secret ingredient!)
1 T hot pepper sesame oil
6 c filtered water
2 T sesame seeds

1) Boil filtered water w/ garlic + ginger.
2) While water is heating, chop vegetables.
3) When water comes to a boil, cook noodles according to directions. When there are 2 minutes cooking time left, turn off the heat + add vegetables, green onions + mushrooms.
4) After boiling has definitively stopped, add miso. (You can spoon out a cup of warm water + dissolve miso first in a smaller mixing bowl, before adding to large pot. A spoon or whisk works well for dissolving.) Definitely don't want to boil miso, as this would "cook" it + destroy the beneficial probiotics + enzymes that are so healing + wonderful!
5) After adding miso, add ume plum vinegar, sesame oil, + sesame seeds. Eat + enjoy! Healing, rejuvenative, + delicious.
6) When re-heating leftover soup, make sure to heat on low + not to boil the miso, in order to preserve all the healthy benefits! ;)

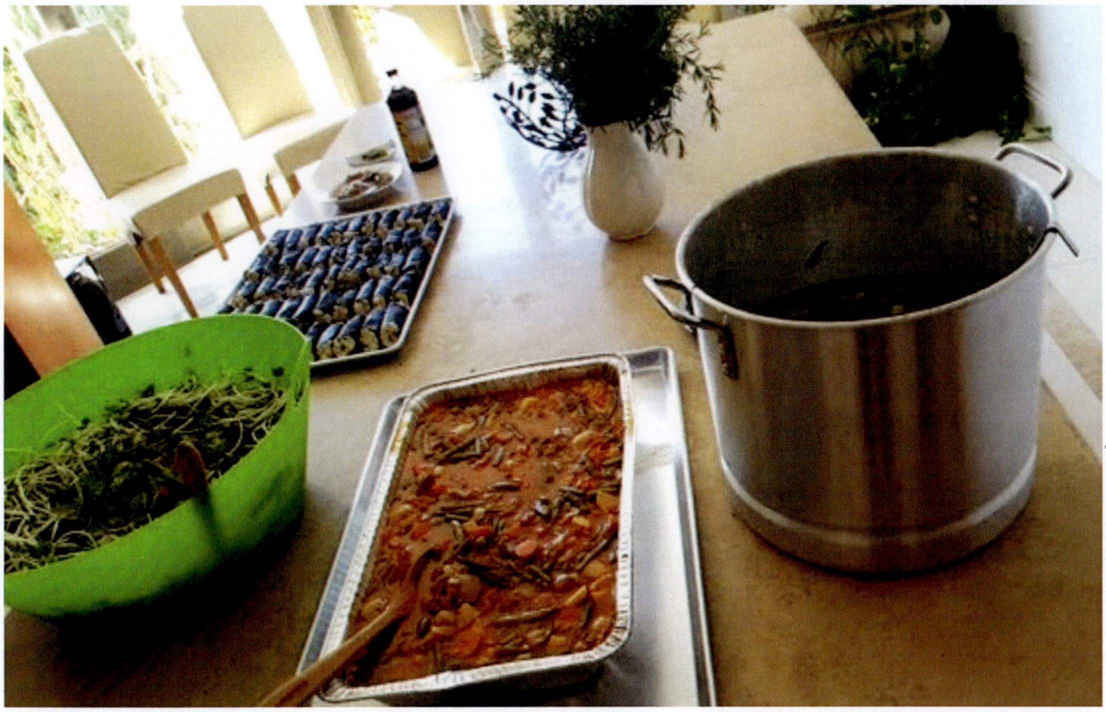

♥Miso-Sesame-Coconut Dressing
Serves: 8
Time: 15 minutes

1 c tahini (can be raw or toasted, I love raw when possible!)
3 T coconut oil
3 T chickpea miso
1/8 c fresh-squeezed lemon juice
4 c filtered water

1) Blend all ingredients together in Vitamix + enjoy!! Yummy poured over leafy green or red leaf lettuce, with cucumber or carrots, it catches the dressing well! ;)

♥Green Salad
Serves: 4
Time: 15 minutes

1 head Leafy Green/ or Red Leaf Lettuce
1 large cucumber, sliced thin
3 carrots, shredded in food processor

1) Wash lettuce + break into bite-size pieces
2) Shred carrots in food processor. Chop cucumber into thin slices.
3) Arrange salad + enjoy with Miso-Sesame-Coconut Dressing!!

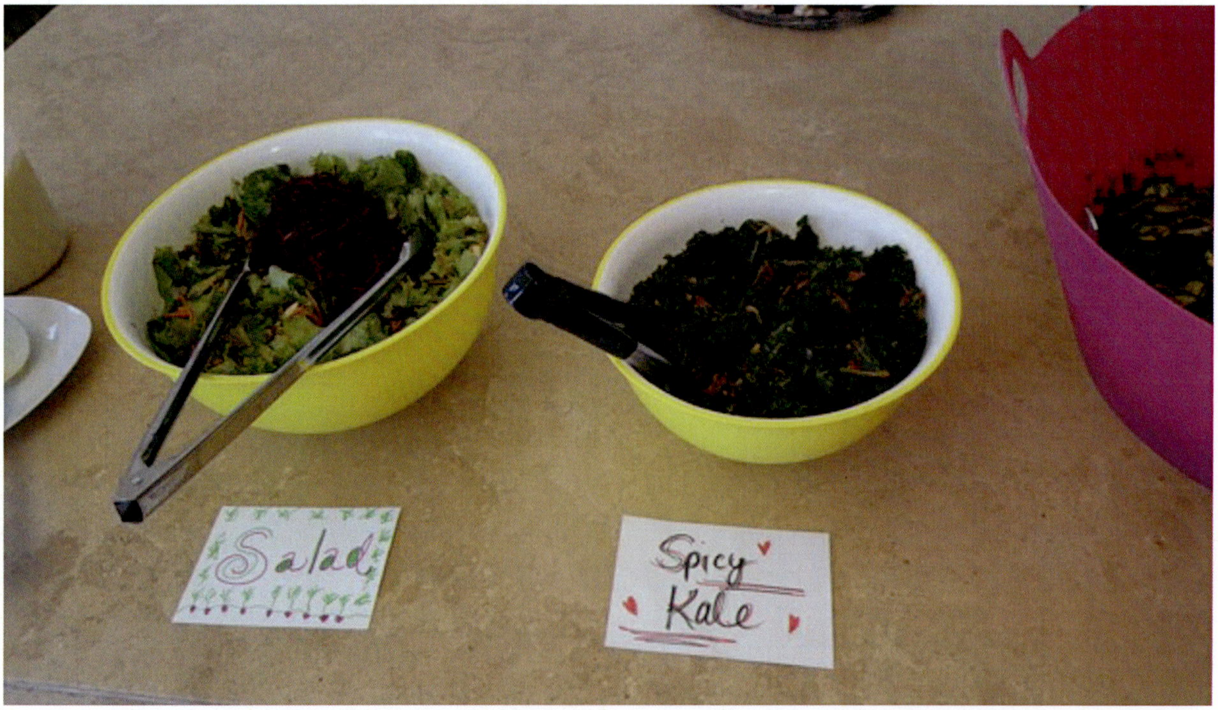

♥Lemon Coconut Pudding

Serves: 4
Time: 35 minutes

1 can coconut milk
2 T fresh-squeezed lemon juice
2 T Grade B maple syrup
½ tsp vanilla extract
pinch sea salt
¼ c chia seeds
1/2 fresh lemon, sliced/ or zested for decoration

1) Blend everything together, except chia seeds + fresh lemon for decoration.
2) When pudding is blended, stir in chia seeds evenly + let sit for 20 minutes. Stir once or twice in between, to make sure chia is soaking up pudding evenly.
3) When chia has "gelled" the pudding, pour into pudding cups + decorate with lemon slices or lemon zest!

♥Sweet Orange Coconut Pudding (a variation of the Lemon Coconut Pudding above!)

Serves: 4
Time: 35 minutes

1 can coconut milk
¼ c chia seeds
1 T raw local honey
½ tsp vanilla extract
1 orange, juiced
½ orange, sliced or zested for decoration

1) Blend everything together, except chia seeds + ½ orange for decoration.
2) When pudding is blended, stir in chia seeds evenly + let sit for 20 minutes. Stir once or twice in between, to make sure chia is soaking up pudding evenly.
3) When chia has "gelled" the pudding, pour into pudding cups + decorate with orange slices or orange zest!

Seasonal Delight Lunch

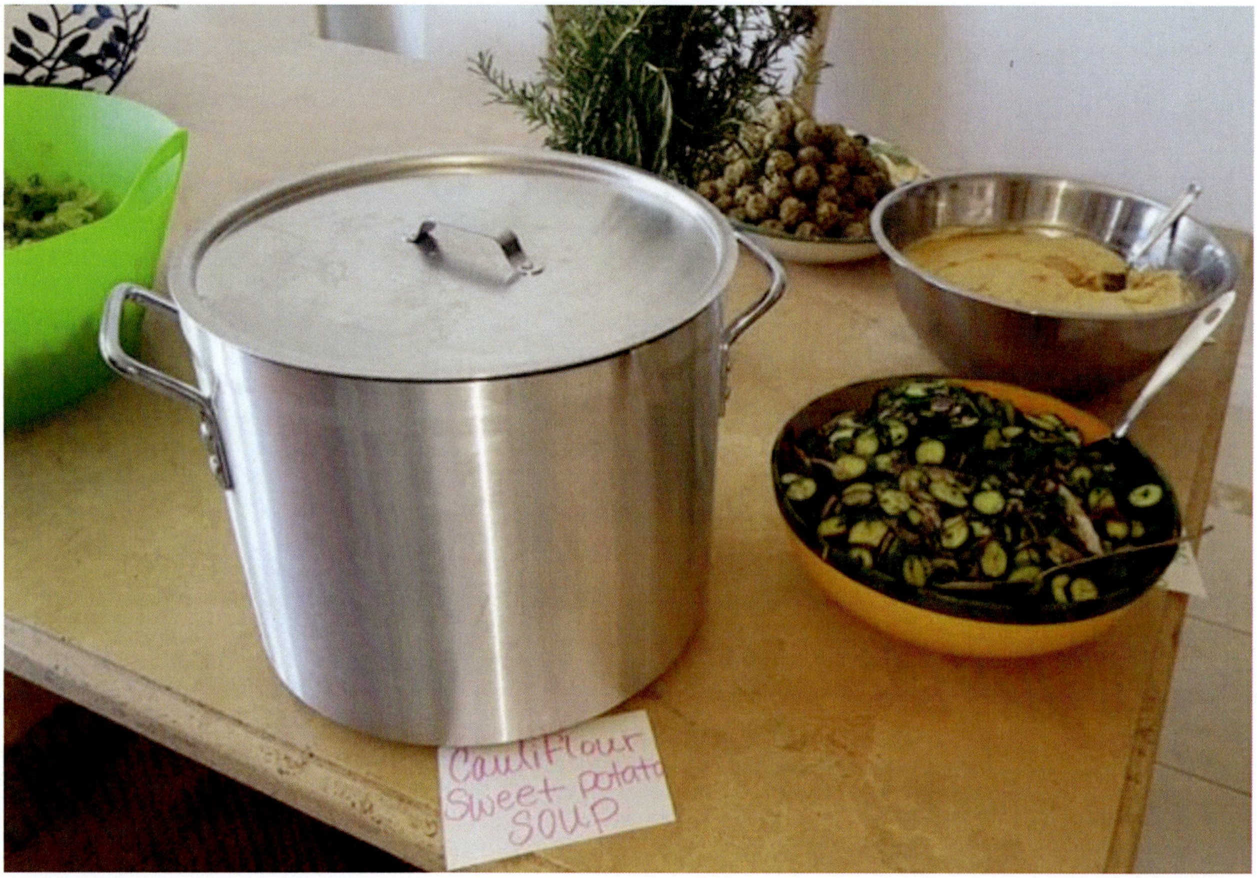

Cauliflower Sweet Potato Soup
Serves: 10
Time: 1 hour

2 large Japanese sweet potatoes, cut into "chunks"
1 large head cauliflower, cut into "chunks"
1 medium yellow onion, minced/ diced
6 carrots, cut into "chunks"
2 T coconut oil
1 large clove garlic, pressed/ minced
2 sprigs fresh rosemary (optional), taken off stem
1 T sea salt
filtered water, enough to cover all ingredients

1) Place potatoes, cauliflower, carrots, + rosemary, into a cooking pot. Cover with filtered water, add a pinch of sea salt, + bring to a boil.
2) Meanwhile, sauté onion + garlic in coconut oil until translucent. When cooked, add to soup pot. (Ingredients can simply be added to cooking pot, but sautéing will give them more flavor.)
3) Once soup ingredients come to a boil, bring heat down to low + cook until potatoes are soft when you stick a fork in them. ;)
4) Now soup is completely cooked. All that's left to do is blend! Batch by batch, ladle soup into the Vitamix/ blender + blend until smooth. Transfer to a new serving pot. When all soup is blended, serve + enjoy!!! This is a great comfort food + winter soup!

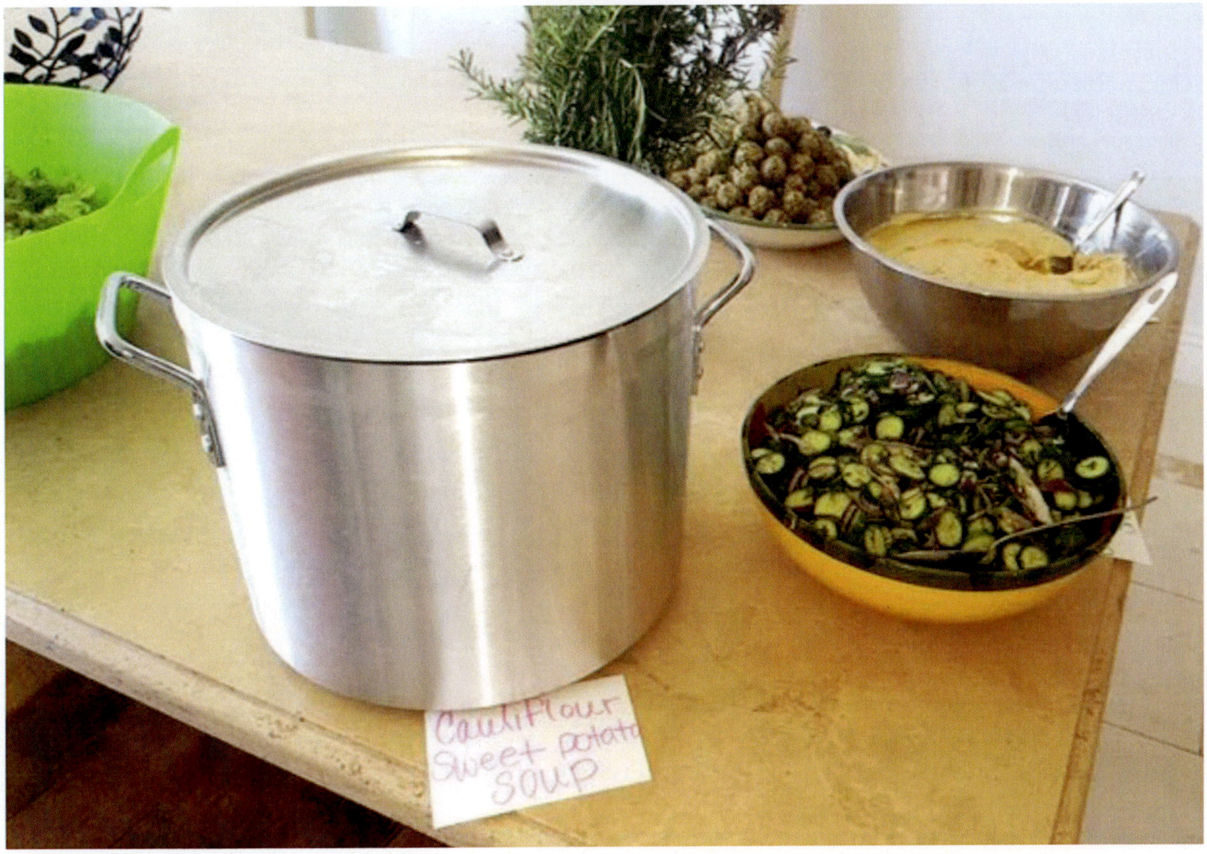

Almond Quinoa
Serves: 5
Time: 30 minutes

1 c Quinoa, dry
2 c filtered water
¼ c slivered almonds
¼ c fresh parsley, chopped finely
1 tsp cumin powder
2 tsp cinnamon powder
½ tsp sea salt

1) Cook quinoa in filtered water, with sea salt, bringing to a boil + then simmering on low until fully cooked (about 20 minutes).
2) Add finely chopped fresh parsley, almonds, + spices, + stir till thoroughly mixed. Add Reiki energy healing love, of course. ;)
3) Yum Yum! Spoon out + enjoy! This is a great base or side dish!

Roasted Broccoli
Serves: 5
Time: 40 minutes

1 large head broccoli, cut into "chunks"/ bite-size florets (you can also use the broccoli stem. Just shave off the tougher outside, then cut the tender inside into "chunks" as well. ;)
3 T olive oil
2 cloves fresh garlic, pressed/ minced
1 tsp sea salt
½ tsp black pepper or pinch cayenne

1) Cut broccoli + place in a mixing bowl. Add pressed garlic, olive oil, sea salt + pepper. Toss/ marinate the broccoli with your loving hands, massaging olive oil into the broccoli.
2) Spread broccoli on olive oil-ed sheet pan + bake @ 350 degrees for 25 minutes or until broccoli starts to smell amazing, + you can stick a fork in it! ;) Yum!

♥Green Salad

Serves: 4
Time: 15 minutes

1 bunch Red Leaf Lettuce
½ large Cucumber, sliced thin
1 ripe tomato, cut into bite-size “chunks”

1) Wash lettuce + cut/ tear into bite-size pieces. Arrange in salad bowl.
2) Add other vegetable decorations/ ingredients, adding more items you love, such as carrots, olives, sprouts, etc.
3) Enjoy with one of the AMAZING salad dressings in this book! ;)

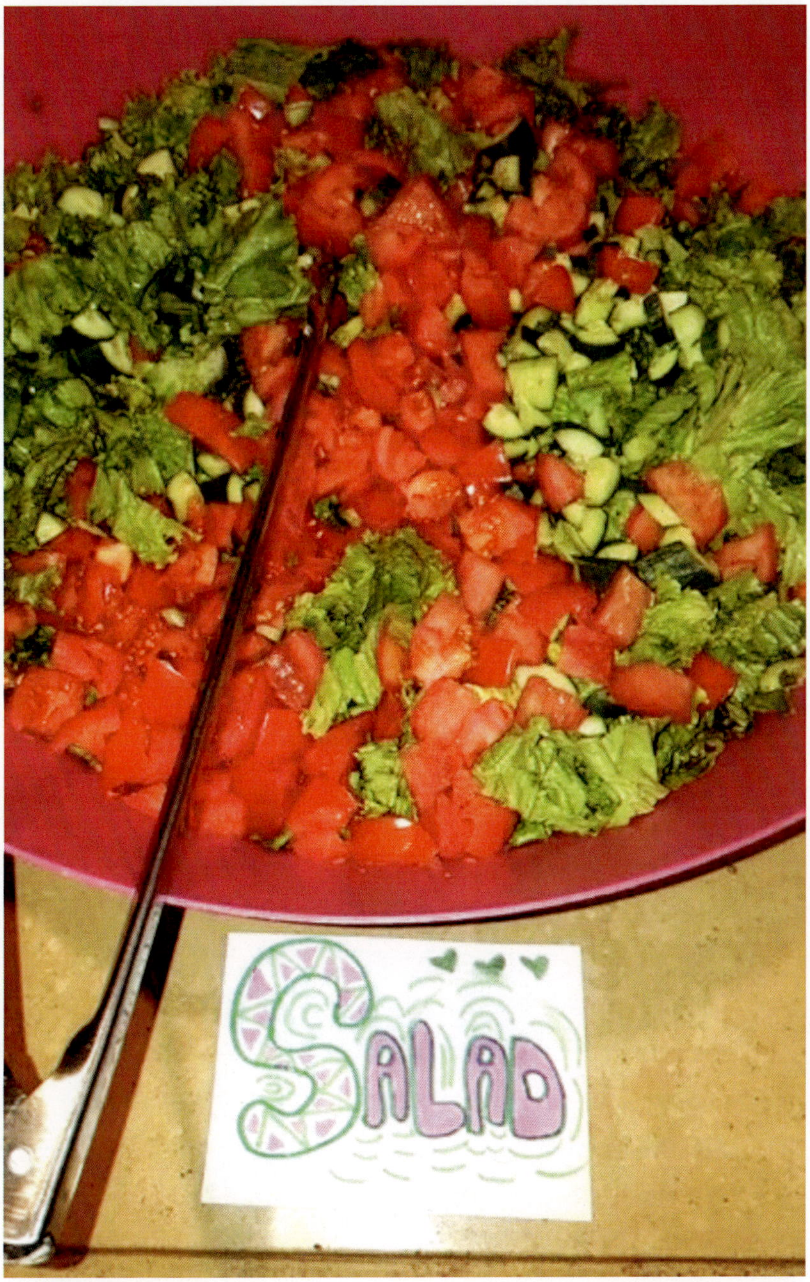

♥∆Cashew Ranch Dressing

Serves: 15 (great to save for 2-3 days!)
Time: 15 minutes

2 c Cashews, soaked
½ bunch fresh dill OR 2 T dried dill
1/4 c fresh-squeezed lemon juice
1 t sea salt
filtered water

1) Soak cashews overnight. Then drain + rinse cashews.
2) Put all ingredients except filtered water into the blender (Vitamix).
3) Add water up to the 4-cup line.
4) Blend + Enjoy!

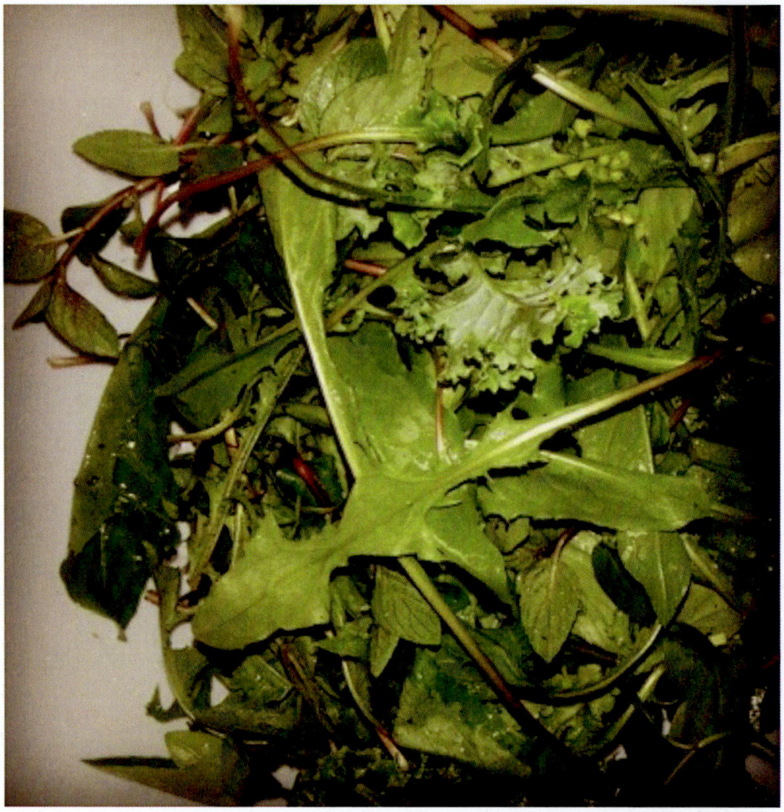

Vegan Enchiladas

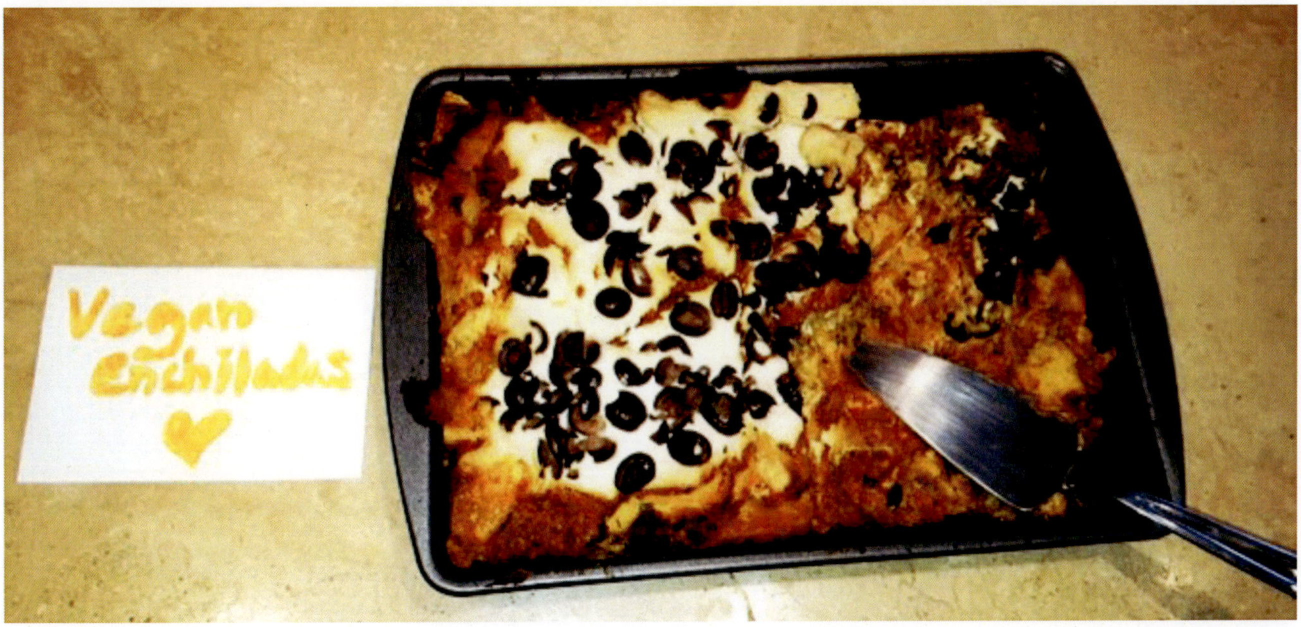

ΔCashew Cheese Kale Enchiladas

Serves: 8
Time: 1 hour

Enchiladas:
1 pack sprouted corn tortillas (I love Ezekiel brand ;))
1 can mild green chiles, chopped (see if you can purchase fresh roasted chiles, or make your own, but for canned, look for preservative-free ;))
1 small can black olives, chopped
1 tomato, diced
1 c vegan red enchilada sauce (see below to make your own! Best b/c sugar-free!)
1 ½ c kale, steamed
cashew cheese (see recipe below)
¼ c fresh cilantro, finely chopped

Cashew Cheese:
1 c cashews, soaked
1 tsp fresh-squeezed lemon juice
¼ tsp chipotle powder (optional)
¼ tsp sea salt
pinch black pepper
1 c filtered water (use only as much as you need to create desired consistency, the more "solid" the better for this recipe ;))

Enchilada Sauce:
1 T olive oil
1 yellow onion, finely chopped
3 cloves garlic, pressed/ minced
1 handful cherry tomatoes
1 2-oz bag dried Ancho chilis (Melissa's brand carries these ;))
1 ½ c filtered water
1 can fire roasted tomatoes (I like Muir Glen organic, you can actually buy these @ Costco ;))
¼ c apple cider vinegar
2 T chickpea flour
3 T chili powder
1 tsp cumin
pinch sea salt

1) Blend together all ingredients in cashew cheese recipe; pour into a bowl + rinse the blender!
2) Blend together all ingredients for Enchilada sauce; pour into a separate bowl.
3) Under "Enchiladas" ingredients, steam kale, chop cilantro, chilis + olives, dice tomato.
4) Next is the fun part! In a glass pan, arrange enchiladas! Curl tortillas with chilis, olives, tomato, kale, cilantro. Drizzle enchilada sauce + cashew cheese inside. Layer curled tortillas in rows, in the glass pan. Pour enchilada sauce + cheese over the whole casserole dish! Yum!
5) Bake at 350 degrees for 20 minutes. Then enjoy! Yum YUM!!!!

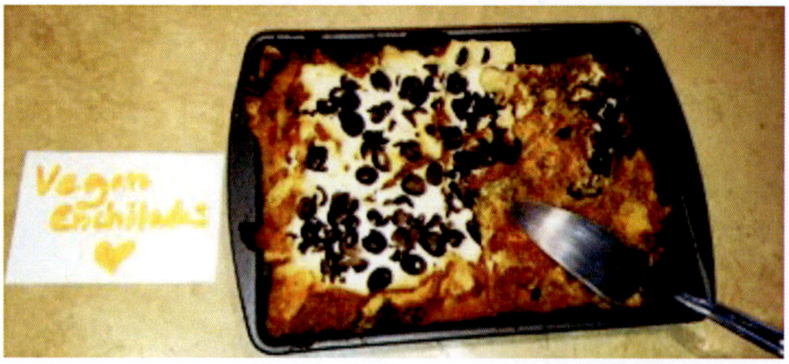

ΔBlack Beans

Serves: 8
Time: 1 hour (requires overnight soaking of beans)

2 c dry black beans (5 cups cooked)
1 tsp sea salt
2 cloves garlic
½ medium yellow onion, finely chopped
1 tomato
1 tsp cumin powder

1) Soak black beans overnight, drain + rinse.
2) Cook w/ filtered water about 4 inches above beans, with a pinch of sea salt, onions + pressed/ minced garlic!
3) Bring to a boil (on high), then reduce heat, add tomatoes, cumin powder + continue to cook until beans are soft. Optional: Add a splash of olive oil for flavor!
4) Enjoy!!

ΔCoconut Brown Rice

Serves: 6
Time: 45 minutes – 1 hour (requires overnight soaking of brown rice)

1 c Brown Rice, dry
1/3 c shredded coconut
1/3 tsp sea salt
1 T coconut oil
1/8 tsp cinnamon
1 pinch cayenne
2 ½ c water

1) Soak rice overnight, rinse + drain.
2) Cook 2 parts water/ 1 part soaked rice, on high. Add a lil sea salt. Bring to a boil, turn down to low until cooked.
3) When rice is cooked, stir in all other ingredients, mix well, + serve! Yum!

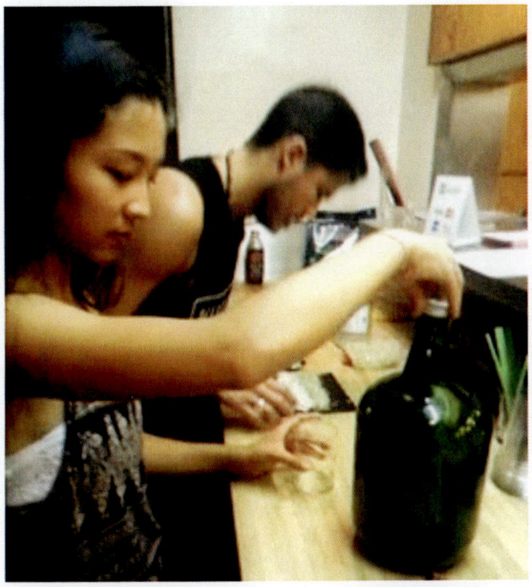

Shakti Mayumi doubles as a sound healer, but she is known to rock it in the kitchen!

♥Romaine Salad w/ Lemon-Olive Oil Dressing

Serves: 4
Time: 15 minutes

1 bunch Romaine Lettuce
¼ bunch Cilantro
3 Carrots/ or 1 daikon radish, shredded
1 T fresh-squeezed lemon juice
1 T olive oil
1/8 tsp sea salt
pinch black pepper

1) Wash + chop Romaine into bite-size pieces. Prepare shredded carrots/ daikon in food processor. Chop cilantro. Place all ingredients into a mixing bowl.
2) Add Lemon juice, olive oil, sea salt + pepper. Toss lovingly into salad. Enjoy!

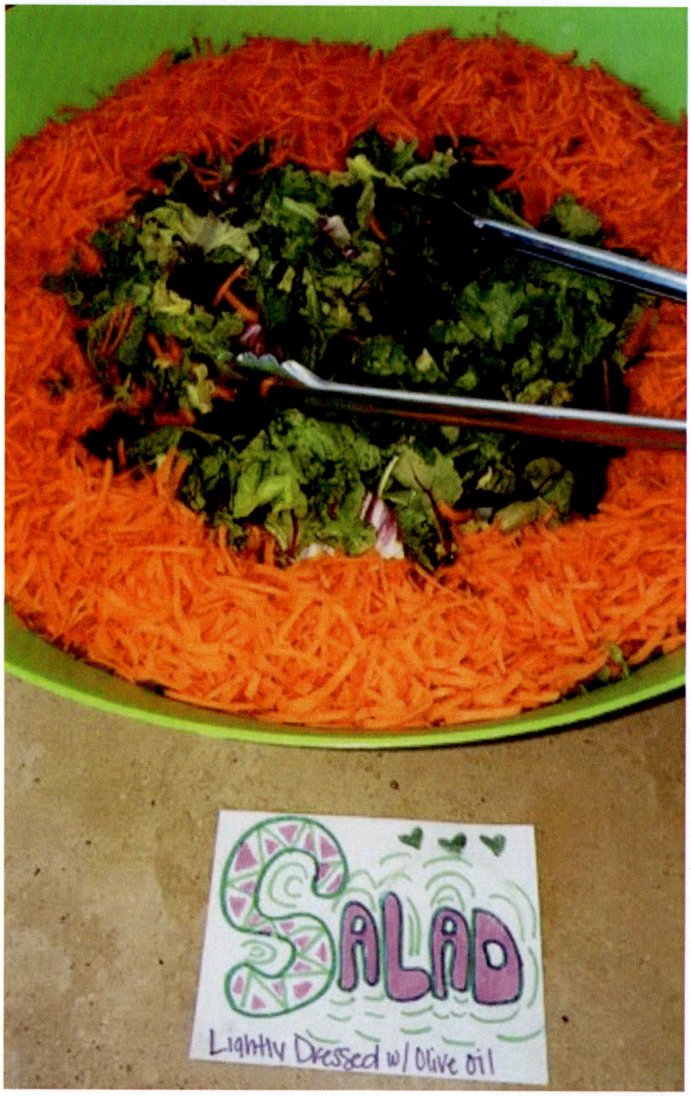

Chickpea Patty Day aka. Winter Goddess

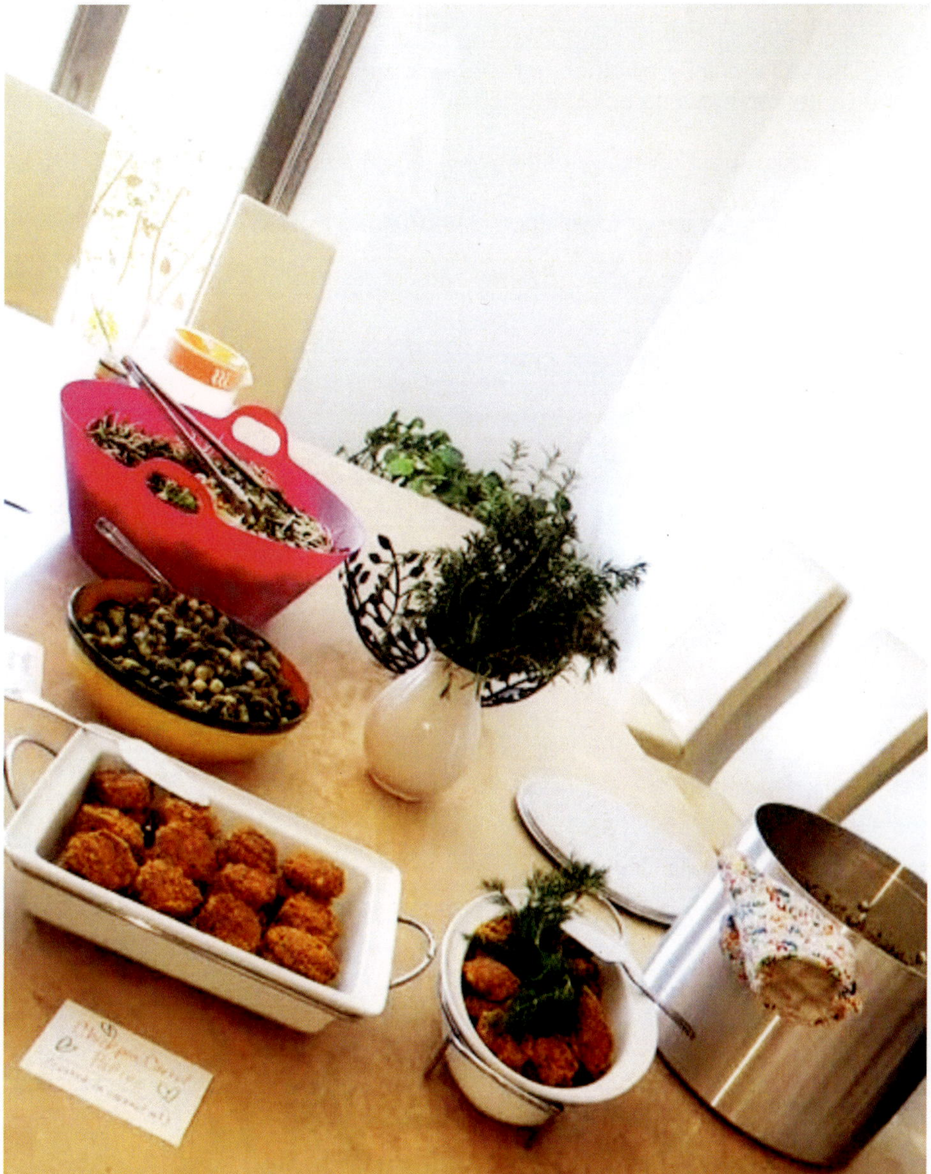

ΔChickpea Patties

Serves: 6
Time: 1 hour 30 minutes (including chickpea cooking time, requires overnight soaking of chickpeas ;))

2 c chickpeas, cooked
4 carrots
½ c Tahini
¼ bunch Parsley
1 tsp cumin powder
1 tsp turmeric powder
1 pinch cayenne
¼ tsp Sea Salt
¼ c coconut oil, for cooking!

1) Soak chickpeas overnight, rinse + drain. Then cook chickpeas with a pinch of sea salt. Drain + cool.
2) In food processor, process fresh parsley till chopped. Then add carrots + chop. Then add chickpeas + process. Then add tahini + all other ingredients, except for coconut oil.
3) Place chickpea patty mixture into a mixing bowl. Mix together + roll in balls/ flatten into patty shapes.
4) Heat coconut oil in a frying pan + heat chickpea patties until brown + crispy on both sides. Flip to cook each side.
5) Place chickpea patties on an organic paper towel-lined plate to drain excess oil (I learned this from my Jewish latke-frying relatives! ;)) Enjoy!!

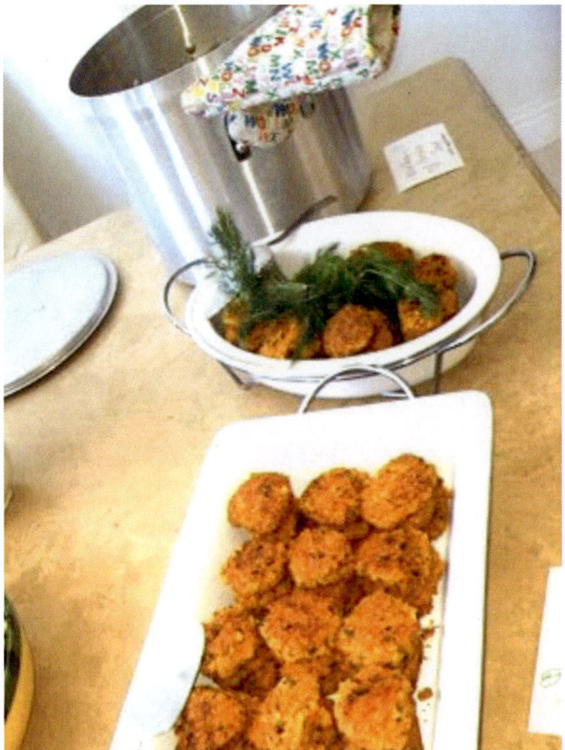

Roasted Brussel Sprouts
Serves: 5
Time: 30 minutes

1 lb Brussel Sprouts
¼ c olive oil
1 tsp sea salt
½ tsp ground black pepper

1) Wash Brussel sprouts + place in a mixing bowl. Drizzle with olive oil, sea salt + pepper. Marinate + massage oil into the Brussel sprouts till all is mixed + well-coated.
2) Pour into an olive oil – greased baking sheet + bake in the oven at 350 degrees for 20 minutes or until crispy on the outside/ slightly browned/ soft on the inside + you can stick a fork in it! Enjoy!!! Healthy + Yum!

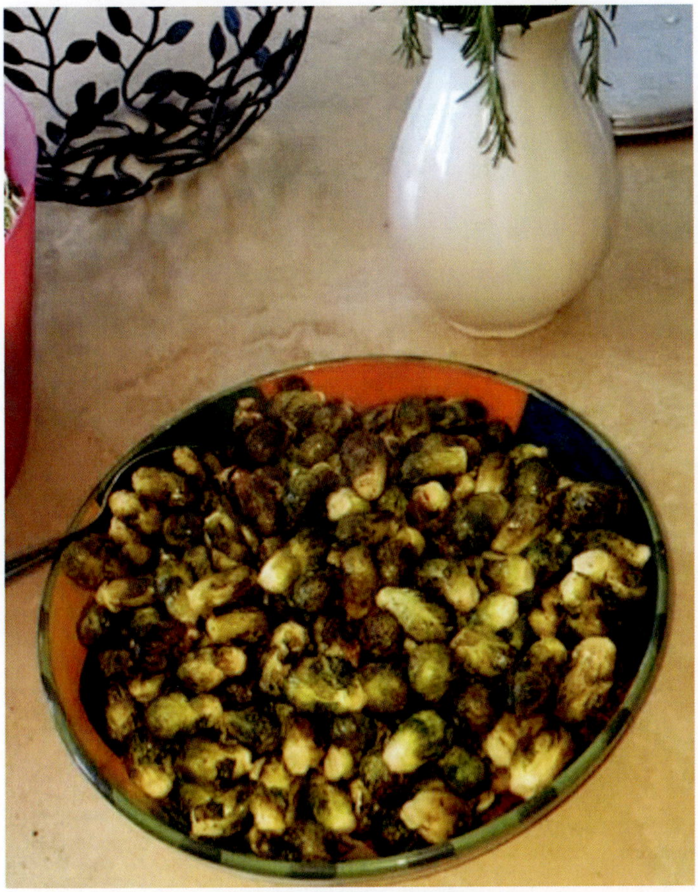

∆Wild Rice – Parsnip Soup

Serves: 6
Time: 40 minutes (requires overnight soaking of wild rice ;))

1 c wild rice, dry
1 c parsnip, cut into bite-size "chunks"
2 T coconut oil
1/3 c onion, minced
½ c celery, chopped finely
2 cloves garlic, pressed/ minced
1 c button mushrooms, sliced
1 tsp black pepper
2 tsp sea salt
2 T fresh sage, finely chopped
5 c filtered water
2 c coconut milk, canned
1 c nutritional yeast

1) This recipe is actually super yummy! Soak wild rice overnight, drain + rinse.
2) Place in a pot to boil: wild rice, parsnip. Cover with filtered water + turn heat to high.
3) Meanwhile heat a pan with coconut oil + heat: onion, garlic, mushrooms + celery. When onion is translucent, pour all these items into the soup pot.
4) When soup pot comes to a boil, turn heat down to low. Then add: sea salt, black pepper, nutritional yeast, fresh sage, + coconut milk. Taste + adjust to your fancy.
5) When wild rice is soft + parsnips are soft in the middle, the soup is done! Eat + enjoy! A hearty yummy winter comfort food! Delicious! Wild Rice, Coconut Milk, + Mushrooms pair well together! ;)

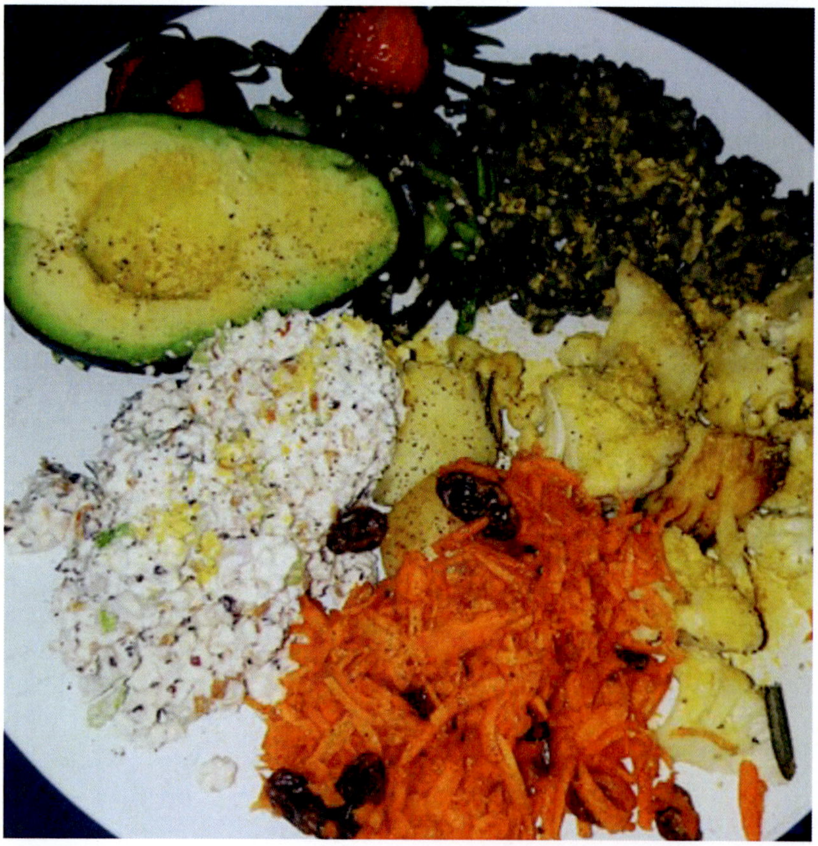

♥Green Salad w/ Citrus – Olive Oil Dressing

Serves: 4
Time: 15 minutes

1 head romaine lettuce
3 carrots, shredded
½ small beet, shredded
1/5 bunch parsley, finely chopped
1 T olive oil
2 T fresh-squeezed orange juice
1 tsp fresh thyme/ or oregano
pinch sea salt

1) Wash + chop romaine lettuce into bite-size pieces. Shred carrot + beet in the food processor. Chop parsley. Toss ingredients into a mixing bowl.
2) Add olive oil, orange juice, dried herbs + sea salt. Mix together with your loving hands. Serve!

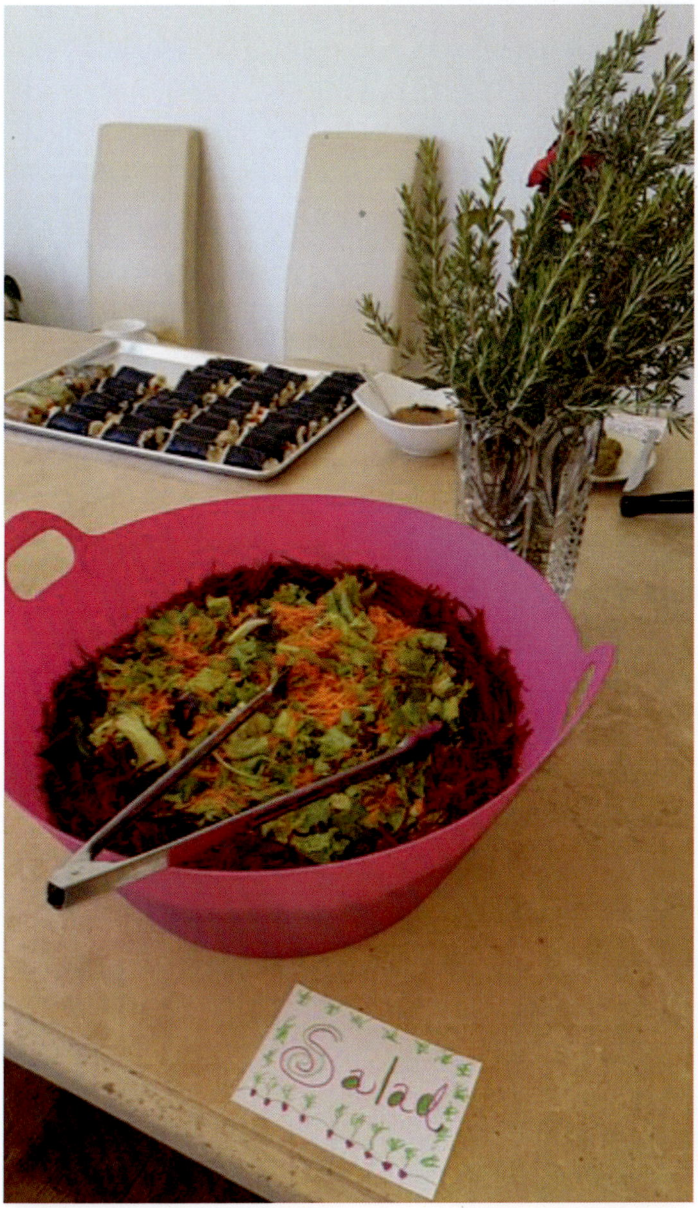

Strawberries + Crème!

((Serve w/ a carton of Fresh, Local Strawberries!))

♥Coconut Crème

Serves: 5
Time: 15 minutes

Meat of 4-5 young coconuts OR 1 ½ cans coconut milk
1/3 c raw local honey OR Grade B maple syrup
1 capful vanilla extract
pinch sea salt
filtered water/ coconut water to desired consistency

1) Blend all ingredients in Vitamix/ blender, adding water/ coconut water a little at a time to keep crème thick, but still well-blended. Yum Yum! Enjoy!

ΔCashew Whipped Crème (an alternative to Coconut Crème above!)

Serves: 4
Time: 20 minutes (requires overnight soaking of cashews)

1 c Cashews, soaked
1 ½ c almond OR coconut milk
¼ c Grade B maple syrup
1 t vanilla extract
pinch sea salt
1 ½ T sunflower lecithin (I love Blue Mountain Organics brand. This is a substitute for soy lecithin, for those who wish to be soy-free!)
1/3 c coconut oil, melted

1) Soak cashews overnight, drain + rinse.
2) Place all ingredients in blender, EXCEPT sunflower lecithin + coconut oil. Blend these first ingredients together.
3) When blended, add sunflower lecithin + coconut oil, last, to thicken Cashew Whipped Crème!
4) Eat with Strawberries, use to top a cake, ice cream, or any fruit or dessert. Yum Yum Yum! And it's vegan! And healthy! Enjoy!!!

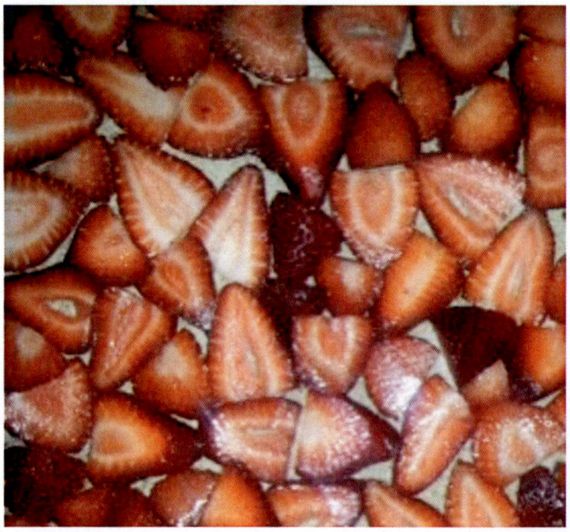

Indian Food

I have a special love for Indian Food, as I spent a semester abroad in Mysore, South India, doing the School for International Training's Gender + Development Program, way back in 1999. I was vegetarian back then, and LOVED that in India, vegetarian food was the norm! The food was AMAZING! And it was one of the things I missed, when going 100% raw.

I am so grateful for Indian Food (I never got sick of it while spending 4 ½ months in India!) I also acknowledge, as with all these world cuisines, I have much more to learn! ;) Visit your local vegetarian Indian food restaurant for a special treat!! ;)

And I have more stories to come, about spending a month at Auroville Community in Tamil Nadu.

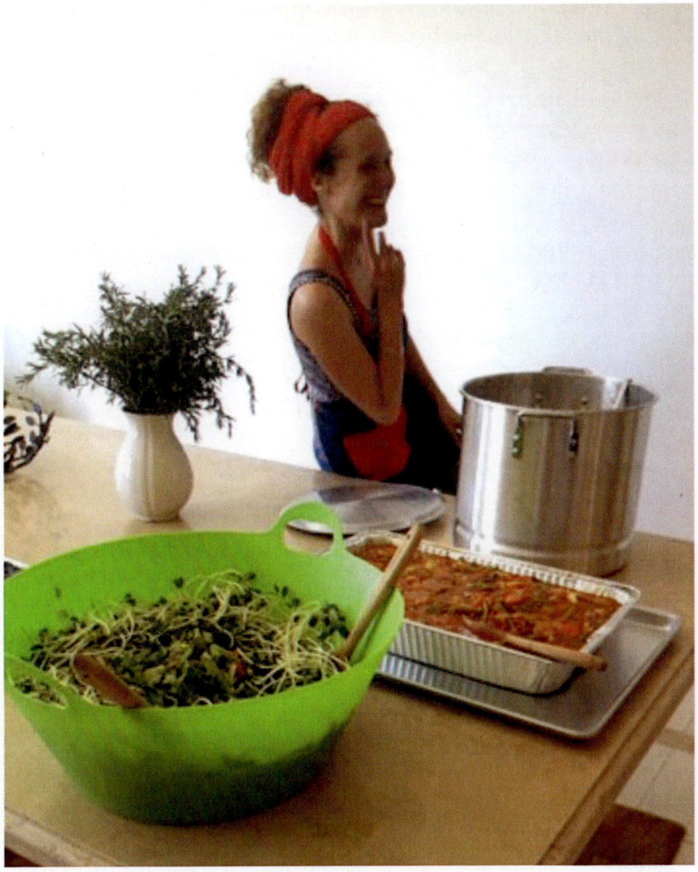

ΔIndian Chana Masala

Serves: 8
Time: 1 ½ hours (requires overnight soaking of chickpeas)

2 T coconut oil
1 c onion
2 cloves garlic, pressed/ minced
1 T ginger, minced
2 c tomato, cut in bite-size "chunks"
1 c dry chickpea, soaked overnight + cooked
2 c water
1 T fresh-squeezed lemon juice
1 T fresh cilantro, finely chopped
1 tsp ground coriander
2 tsp ground cumin
½ tsp fennel seeds
1 tsp garam masala
1 tsp sea salt
4 whole cloves
2 cardamom pods

1) Soak chickpeas overnight w/ filtered water. Use 2-3 times as much water as chickpeas, as they will expand to soak up all the water!
2) The next day, drain water from chickpeas, + rinse 2-3 times with running water, to remove any residue + keep the beans fresh + easily digestible! Ideally the 3rd time, the water will run clear + they are ready to cook!
3) Cook chickpeas in filtered water (again, twice as much water as chickpeas) along with a pinch of sea salt/ pink Himalayan salt.
4) Meanwhile in a separate pan, heat up coconut oil + sauté chopped onion, pressed garlic, finely chopped ginger, along with whole spices: fennel, clove + cardamom. Heat until the onion is clear.
5) When chickpeas come to a boil, add sautéed ingredients, along with cumin, coriander + garam masala. Also add tomato + continue to cook on low heat until chickpeas are soft (up to 45 minutes).
6) Right before serving, add cilantro + lemon juice, + serve! Yum!

ΔSpinach Dahl – inspired by Vegan Richa's Dal Fry Spiced Indian Lentil Soup, VeganRicha.com
Serves: 4
Time: 1-1 ½ hours

½ c red lentils
3 ½ c filtered water
2 tsp coconut oil
½ tsp cumin seeds
½ tsp black mustard seeds (if you can't find, use yellow mustard seeds ;))
1 hot green chili
1 c yellow onion, finely chopped
1 tsp ground coriander
½ tsp turmeric powder
¼ tsp cayenne
1 large tomato, cut in bite-size "chunks"
1 tsp fresh-squeezed lemon juice
¾ tsp sea salt
¼ c cilantro, finely chopped

1) Soak lentils overnight w/ filtered water. Use twice as much water as lentils, as they will expand to soak up all the water!
2) The next day, drain water from lentils, + rinse 2-3 times with running water, to remove any residue + keep the beans fresh + easily digestible! Ideally the 3rd time, the water will run clear + they are ready to cook!
3) Cook lentils in filtered water along with a pinch of sea salt/ pink Himalayan salt.
4) Meanwhile in a separate pan, heat up coconut oil + sauté chopped onion, cumin seeds, mustard seed, + green chili. Heat until the onion is clear.
5) When lentils come to a boil, add sautéed ingredients, along with turmeric powder, coriander, cayenne. Add tomato + continue to cook on low heat until lentils are soft (about 40 minutes).
6) Right before serving, add cilantro + lemon juice, + serve! Yum!

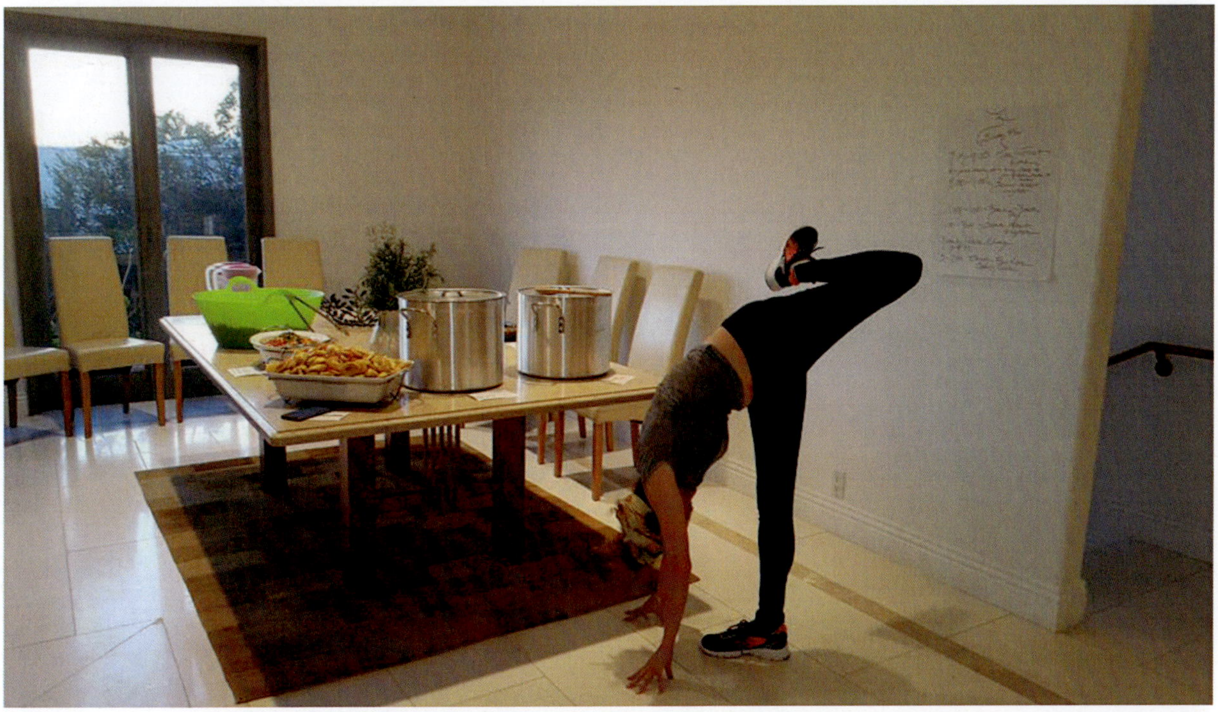

ΔCoriander Biryani Rice - inspired by Coriander Rice Recipe/ Cilantro Rice, VegRecipesofIndia.com

Serves: 3
Time: 1 hour – 1 hour 15 minutes

1 c Brown Rice
2 T coconut oil
1 medium onion, minced
3 cloves garlic, pressed/ minced
½ inch ginger, minced
1 green chili, finely chopped
1 medium potato, cut into chunks
1/3 c green peas (can be organic frozen)
½ c fresh cilantro, finely chopped
2 T shredded coconut
2 cloves
5 black peppers
½ tsp fennel seed
2 cardamom pods
¼ tsp turmeric powder
½ tsp cinnamon
½ tsp cumin powder
1 ½ c filtered water
1/2 tsp sea salt

1) Soak rice overnight, rinse + drain.
2) Cook 2 parts water/ 1 part soaked rice, on high. Add potato chunks + a lil sea salt. Bring to a boil, then turn down to low.
3) Meanwhile, heat coconut oil in a pan + add onion, garlic, ginger, green chili, + whole spices: cloves, black peppers, cardamom pods, fennel seed. Heat until the onion is clear.
4) When rice + potatoes are boiling, turn down to low heat + add all sautéed ingredients, plus ground spices: turmeric, cinnamon, cumin. Add peas + cook till rice is done.
5) When rice is cooked, stir in shredded coconut + cilantro, mix well, + serve! Yum!

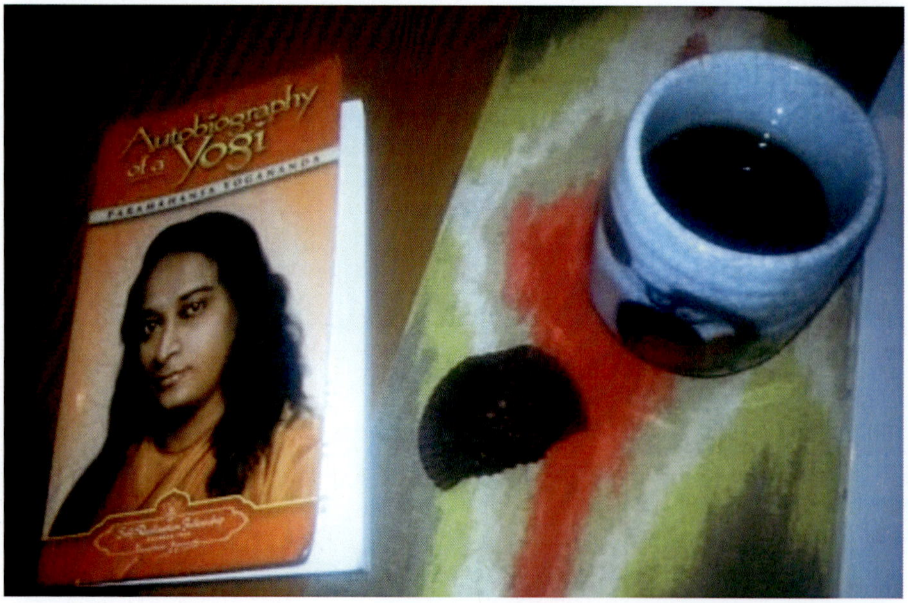

Vegan Aloo Gobi Mutter w/ Green Beans – inspired by Vegan Richa, Vegan Aloo Gobi Mutter
Dad's Favorite, VeganRicha.com
Serves: 6
Time: 45 minutes

2 c potatoes, cut into "chunks"
2 c cauliflower florets (about 1 cauliflower), cut into "chunks"
1 c green peas (can be organic frozen)
1 green chili, finely chopped
1 T garlic, pressed/ minced
2 tsp ginger, minced
1 T coconut oil
1 tsp cumin seeds
¼ tsp cumin powder
¼ tsp turmeric powder
½ tsp coriander
¼ tsp chili powder OR cayenne
2/3 tsp sea salt
1 1/2 c fresh green beans

1) In a pot, steam potatoes, cauliflower, + green beans in an inch of filtered water. Do this by bringing the water to boil on high heat, then turn down to low when water is boiling.
2) Meanwhile, in a pan, heat coconut oil + sauté green chili, garlic + ginger. Add cumin seeds. When these are lightly cooked, add these sautéed ingredients to vegetables.
3) Next add cumin powder, turmeric, coriander, chili/ cayenne, + sea salt. Add peas + cook pot for a few more minutes, until everything is mixed well + yummy!

♥⊕Goat/ Coconut Yogurt Raita w/ Pickle
Serves: 6
Time: 15 minutes

Why goat yogurt? I personally prefer vegan coconut yogurt! But for some, who cannot digest dairy, goat yogurt can be an interesting alternative. Supposedly goat's milk is more digestible than cow's. If you are a dairy eater, goat's milk yogurt may be worth a try. ;)

That, and I am breaking out of labels, into being a Debratarian! And it's so exciting for me to welcome including small amounts of vegetarian, non-vegan alternatives here + there! ;) Thanks for partaking in this experiment! ;)

1 32-oz container goat yogurt/ or plain, unsweetened coconut yogurt
1 large cucumber, sliced in thin "half-moons"
½ red onion, sliced very thin
1 T fresh-squeezed lemon juice
2 sprigs fresh dill, finely chopped
1/4 tsp sea salt
1 jar Indian Lemon Pickles! (can be bought at an Indian grocery store ;))

1) Chop cucumber, onion, dill. Pour yogurt into mixing bowl. Squeeze in lemon, add cucumber, onion, + dill. Add sea salt, + stir everything together.
2) Serve! Pretty! With lemon pickles + plain rice makes a yummy after-dinner finale!

♥ΔRaw Carrot Cake w/ Cashew Crème (an original, vintage Debra Mazer creation ;))
Serves: 15
Time: 1 hour (requires overnight soaking of cashews, sunflower seeds, walnuts, raisins, dates)

Cake:
6 c carrot pulp (save from juicing, + remember to cut off tops + bottoms of carrots first! ;))
1 c soaked sunflower seeds
2 c soaked pitted dates
1 c soaked raisins
1 c soaked walnuts, coarsely chopped
1 T cinnamon
1 tsp ginger powder
1 tsp nutmeg
1 tsp lemon juice

Icing:
2 c soaked cashews
¼ c raw local honey
¼ tsp vanilla extract
pinch sea salt

For Cake:

1) Soak sunflower seeds overnight, drain + rinse. Same with walnuts! Soak raisins + dates separately as well, overnight.
2) Juice carrots + collect the pulp/ or ask your local juice bar to collect theirs for you. ;)
3) Food process everything except the raisins + walnuts, + carrot pulp. It's great to start with sunflower seeds, chop, then add the rest.
4) Fold in raisins, walnuts, + carrot pulp.
5) Line a pie plate w/ plastic wrap + press half the batter in. Flip upside down, + repeat w/ other half, icing in between the layers, + then on outside of cake.

For Icing:

1) Soak cashews overnight, drain + rinse.
2) Blend together all ingredients fur a "butter-cream" cashew frosting!
3) Don't forget to frost in-between, + on top!
4) After the cake is frosted, you may decorate w/ raisins, nuts, currants, shredded coconut, etc.
5) Chill cake for 15 minutes – 1 hour, then cut + serve!

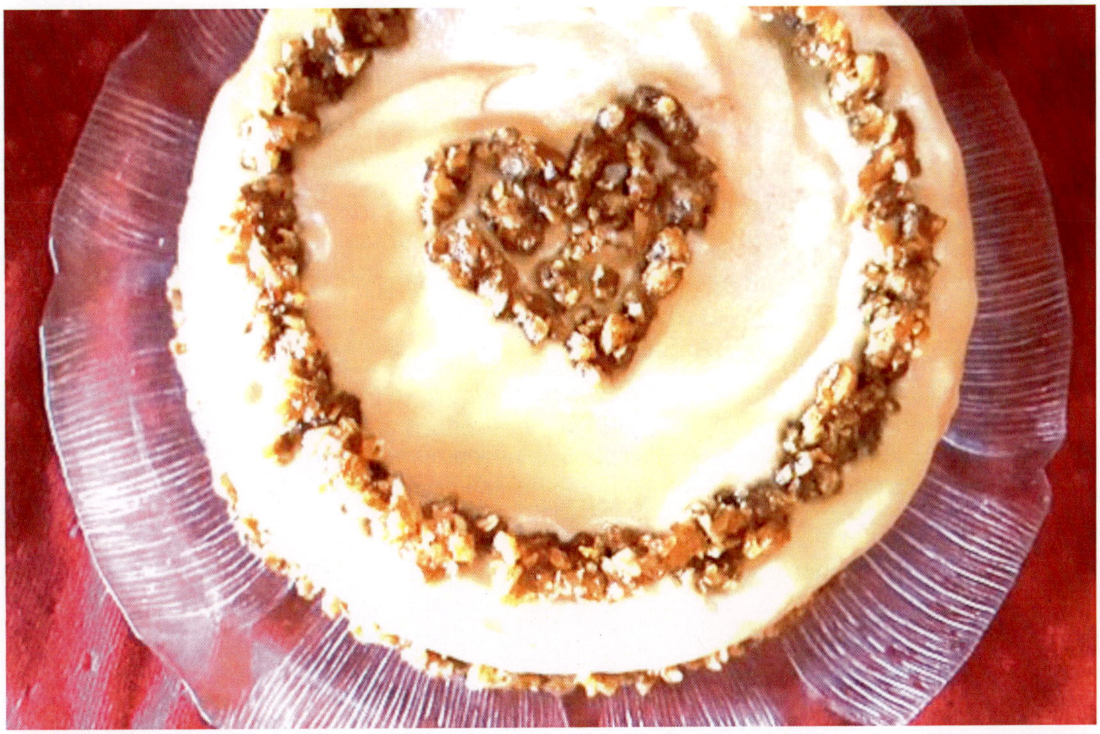

Persian Feast

I have to say, this entire meal was inspired by my Persian friends, Ava Tehrani, Shadi Shariat + Navid Aslani. I know these dishes do not nearly touch the Gloriousness that is Persian food, but it is a start, for me! ;) When I hear these friends are cooking Persian food for holidays or to warm the soul, I wonder, how can I expand myself + learn something new? Thank You Dear Ones! May we all become welcoming to Diversity, in its many gorgeous forms!!! Let this just be the beginning!

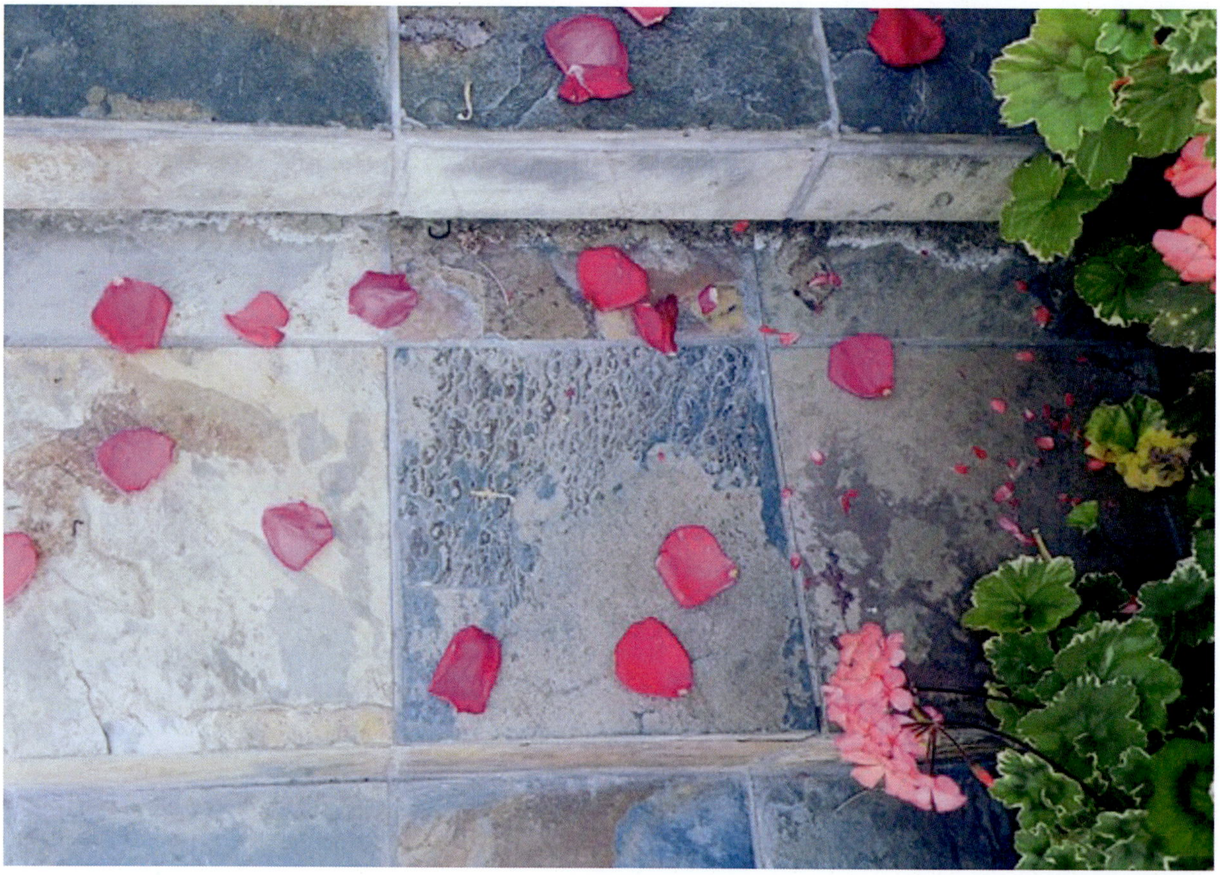

ΔPersian Lentil Stew (Adasi)

Serves: 6
Time: 45 minutes (requires overnight soaking of lentils)

2 c lentils, dry
1 onion, minced
4 cloves garlic, pressed/ minced
1 carrot, chopped into rounds
1 celery stalk, finely chopped
4 T olive oil
6 c filtered water/ or vegetable broth (look for all-natural broth + healthy oils in your vegetable broth!)
1 tsp turmeric
1 tsp cinnamon
2 tsp ground coriander
2 tsp cumin seeds
1 tsp sea salt
1 tsp black pepper
1 lemon, juiced

1) Soak lentils overnight w/ filtered water. Use twice as much water as lentils, as they will expand to soak up all the water!
2) The next day, drain water from lentils, + rinse 2-3 times with running water, to remove any residue + keep the beans fresh + easily digestible! Ideally the 3rd time, the water will run clear + they are ready to cook!
3) Cook lentils in filtered water along with a pinch of sea salt/ pink Himalayan salt.
4) Meanwhile in a separate pan, heat up coconut oil + sauté chopped onion, pressed garlic, carrot, + celery. Heat until the onion is clear.
5) When lentils come to a boil, add sautéed ingredients, along with spices, + continue to cook on low heat until lentils are soft (up to 1 hour).
6) Just before serving, add lemon juice. Enjoy!

Persian Raisin "Jeweled" Quinoa
Serves: 10
Time: 35 - 40 minutes

1 c quinoa
2 c filtered water
2 T sea salt
2 oranges, juiced
1 c raisins, soaked
1 tsp saffron/ or turmeric
2 T coconut oil
1 c sliced almonds/ pistachios
3 carrots, sliced into thin rounds
2 tsp cardamom
2 tsp cinnamon

1) Cook quinoa in filtered water, with carrots, raisins + sea salt, bringing to a boil + then simmering on low until fully cooked (about 20 minutes).
2) Add sliced almonds, spices, orange juice + coconut oil + stir till thoroughly mixed. Add Reiki love, of course. ;)
3) Yum Yum! Spoon out + enjoy! This is a great base or side dish!

♥⊕Kale-Citrus Salad w/ Goat Cheese
Serves: 3
Time: 15 minutes

Again, a note on Goat Cheese! As a dairy lover (if you are) it is interesting to learn that for some, goat's dairy can be more digestible to us humans, than cow's dairy. You can totally leave the Goat Cheese out, on this recipe. Or, if you're feeling daring, and not 100% vegan, put it in!

1 bunch curly green Kale
1 orange, peeled + sliced, into bite-size pieces
1 pinch sea salt
¼ red onion, thinly sliced
1 T olive oil
3 T (spoonfuls) Goat Cheese, preferably organic/ ethically sourced

1) Wash, de-stem, + chop kale into loving bite-size pieces. Place into mixing bowl.
2) Add sliced red onion, sea salt + olive oil, + begin to marinate, massaging kale with loving hands until kale wilts, + each piece is coated with olive oil.
3) Next, add orange bites + toss salad together.
4) Serve individually, topped with goat cheese. Or, serve collectively, with goat cheese to add, on the side. ;) Goes well with Persian dinner! Enjoy!

Chickpea Flour Fudge (Besan Burfi) – inspired by Vegan Richa, Besan Burfi with Condensed Milk Dairy-Free, VeganRicha.com
Serves: 12
Time: 45 minutes

This recipe is entirely made over the stove; no baking! ;) I'm also learning that this recipe is both Indian + Persian in heritage! ;)

2 T coconut oil
1 c chickpea flour
1 c almond milk
½ c coconut palm sugar
2 T ground cashew (fine flour consistency, if possible – you can food process!)
½ c slivered almonds (garnish)
¼ tsp ground cardamom
½ tsp vanilla extract
pinch sea salt

1) Heat 1 T coconut oil (half of what's listed) in a pan + add chickpea flour! Roast the flower over low-medium heat for 10 minutes, until it smells nutty + darkens slightly.
2) In another saucepan, heat other 1 T coconut oil, almond milk, + coconut palm sugar. (You are essentially making vegan condensed milk! ;)) Cook for 10 minutes. Add sea salt + finely ground cashew + whisk together. Boil for another 10 minutes, then take off the heat. Add cardamom + vanilla extract.
3) Next, bring the two sets of ingredients together. Add the roasted flour to the almond milk mixture, + bring back to low heat, whisking away any lumps in the flour. ;)
4) Within a minute or two, the mixture will start to thicken. When the consistency has turned to fudge, drop the mixture into a coconut-oiled pan. Top with slivered almonds to garnish, + cut into squares.
5) Cool + serve! Yummy!

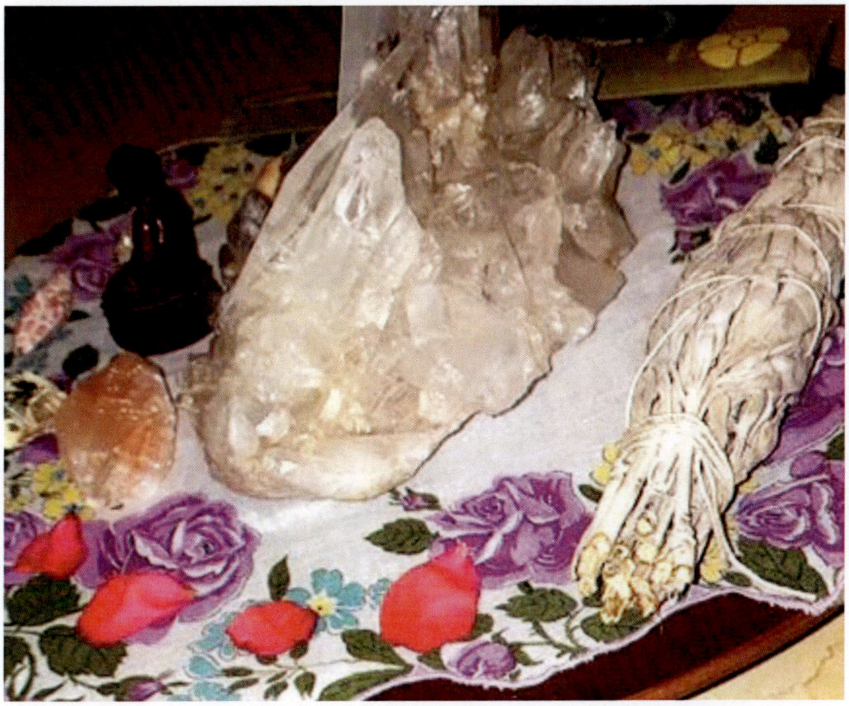

Quinoa Spanish Rice Add-Ons

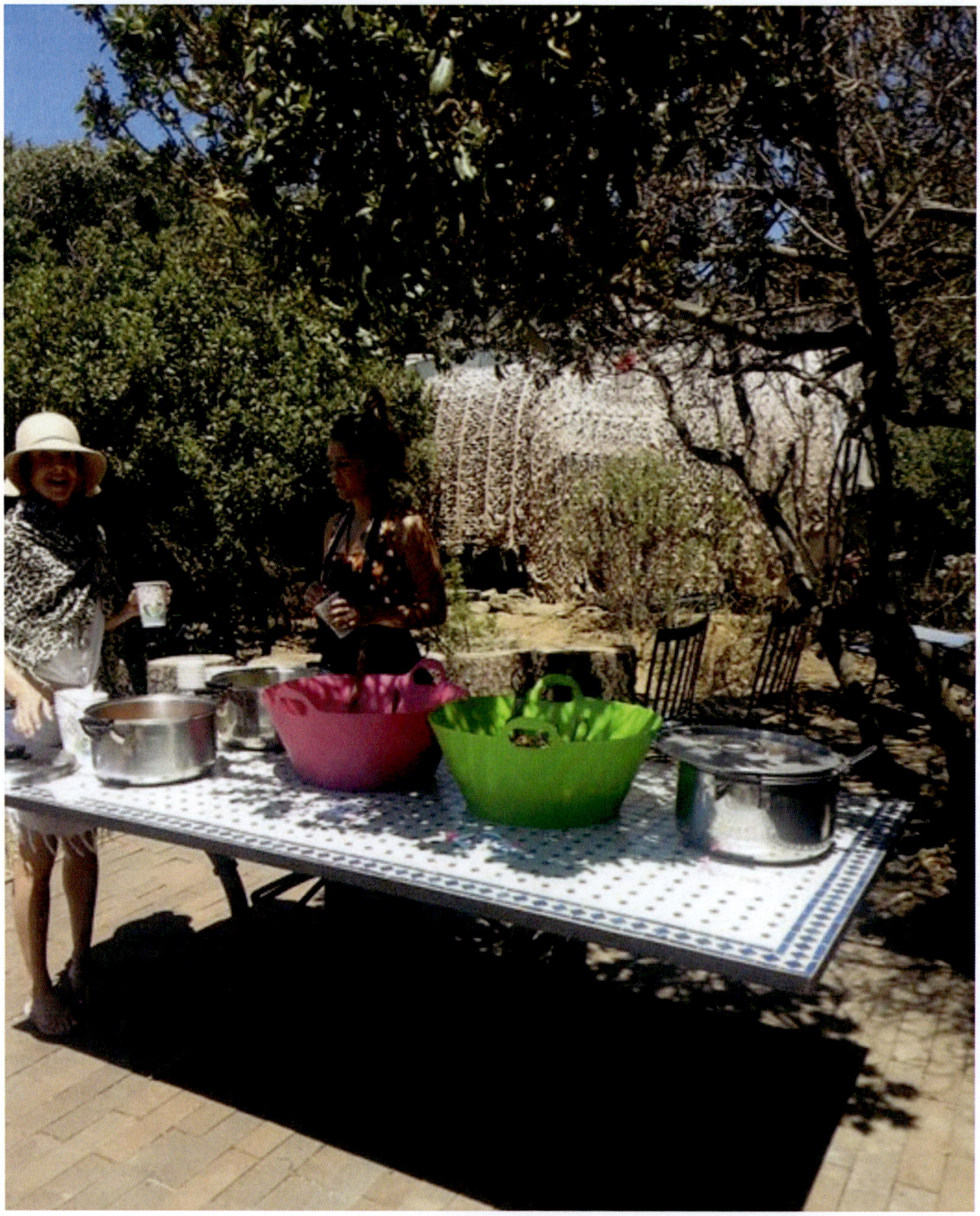

Quinoa Spanish "Rice"
Serves: 6
Time: 45 minutes

This recipe is from our first retreat in Malibu, at Wishtoyo Chumash Village. Such a special + beautiful outdoor cooking + eating experience! With gratitude to all the wonderful Wishtoyo/ Native American folks who welcomed us with open arms, into your circle, your kitchen, and your land. (And even lent me aluminum foil + lit the stove, when I needed it! ;)) Thanks for sharing stories with us, and for your generosity. It was a pleasure + an honor to be there.

1 ½ c quinoa, dry
1 ½ c tomato, cut into "chunks"
1 clove garlic, pressed/ minced
1 small yellow onion, cut into "chunks"
2 1/3 c filtered water
1 large red bell pepper, chopped
1 can green chilis (or fresh roasted chilis are even better!) (look for no citric acid, Bueno Foods is a good brand!)
2 T coconut oil
2 tsp chili powder
1 tsp sea salt

1) Sauté onion, garlic, red bell pepper in coconut oil. Until onion is translucent.
2) Meanwhile begin cooking quinoa w/ filtered water, but include tomato, chilis, spices + sea salt. Add sautéed vegetables when they are ready. Bring quinoa to a boil, then simmer on low.
3) The idea with "Spanish rice" style quinoa is that everything cooks in, marinates + simmers together. When it's ready, enjoy! Delicious, + surprisingly, a great comfort food!

♥Creamy Cabbage Slaw
Serves: 12
Time: 20 minutes

1 large green cabbage
¼ purple cabbage
1 c grapeseed Vegenaise (ooh, this is getting vegan treat-y!)
½ c fresh-squeezed lemon juice
1 T sea salt
3 T olive oil
1/3 bunch fresh cilantro
5 carrots, shredded
6 radishes, shredded, or cut into thin rounds

1) Thinly slice cabbage + place in a large (stainless steel) mixing bowl.
2) Grate carrots + radishes in food processor + add to bowl. (You can also slice radishes if you prefer. ;))
3) Chop cilantro finely + add.
4) Add all other ingredients + stir! You can get in there with your healing Reiki hands + massage everything in! ;)
5) This dish keeps really well! It's easy, yummy + healthy!

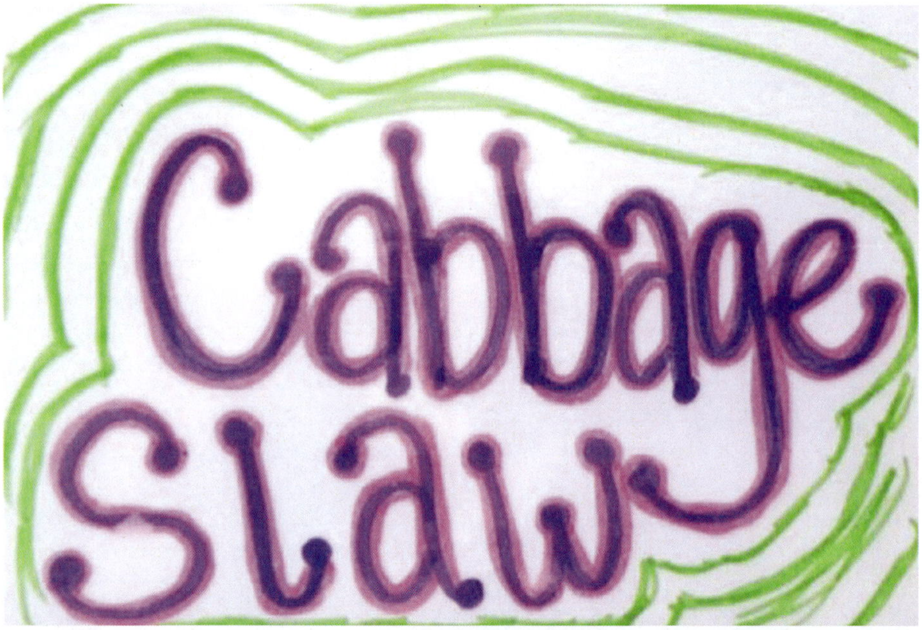
Cabbage
Slaw

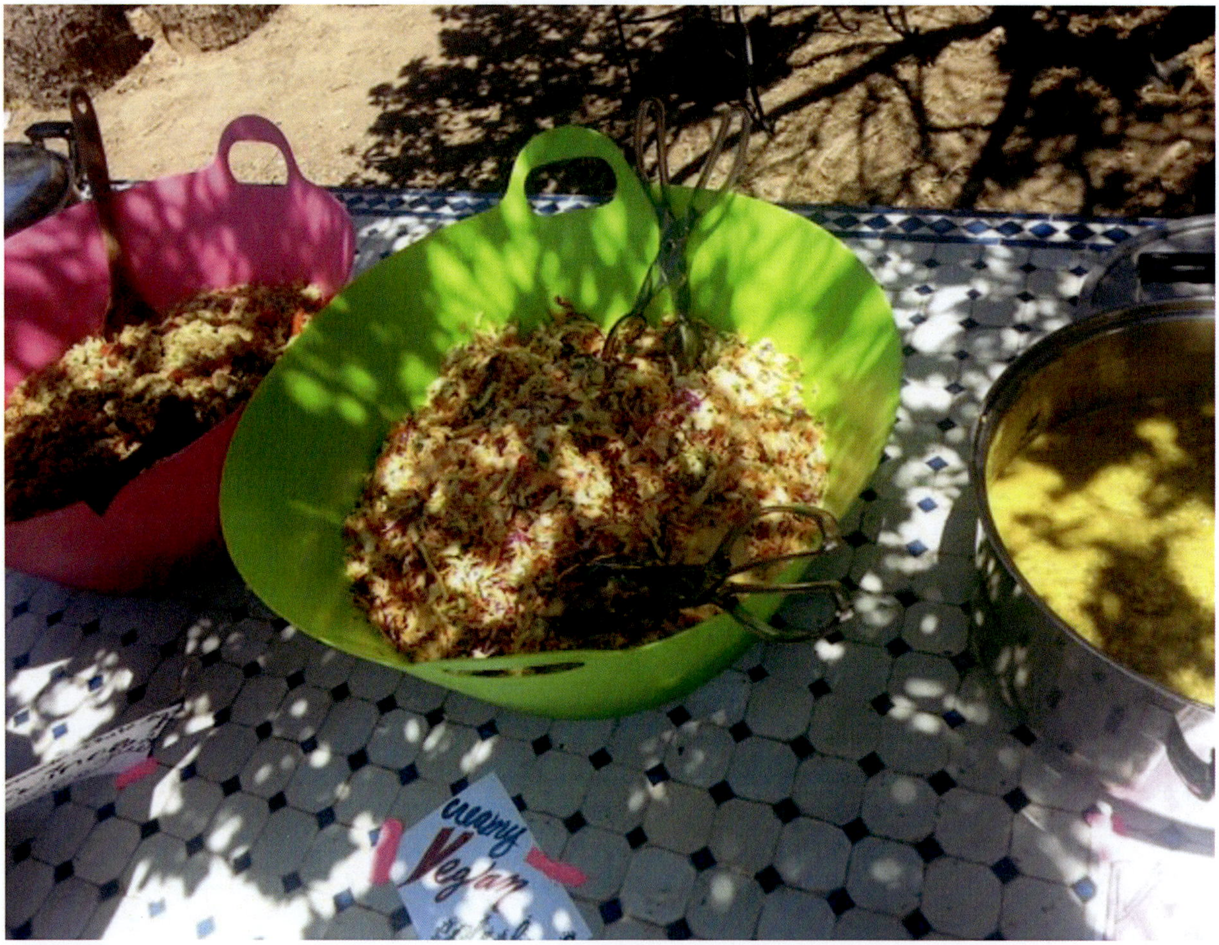
creamy
Vegan

♥Avocado-Lime Dressing

Serves: 10
Time: 15 minutes

1 Reed Avocado (large, or 2 small avocados)
2 limes
1 ½ tsp sea salt
2 T olive oil
1 c filtered water
¼ bunch fresh cilantro

1) Place all items in the blender + blend! (Of course, you'll want to pit + scoop your avocado, juice the lime, + wash the cilantro!) Enjoy!!

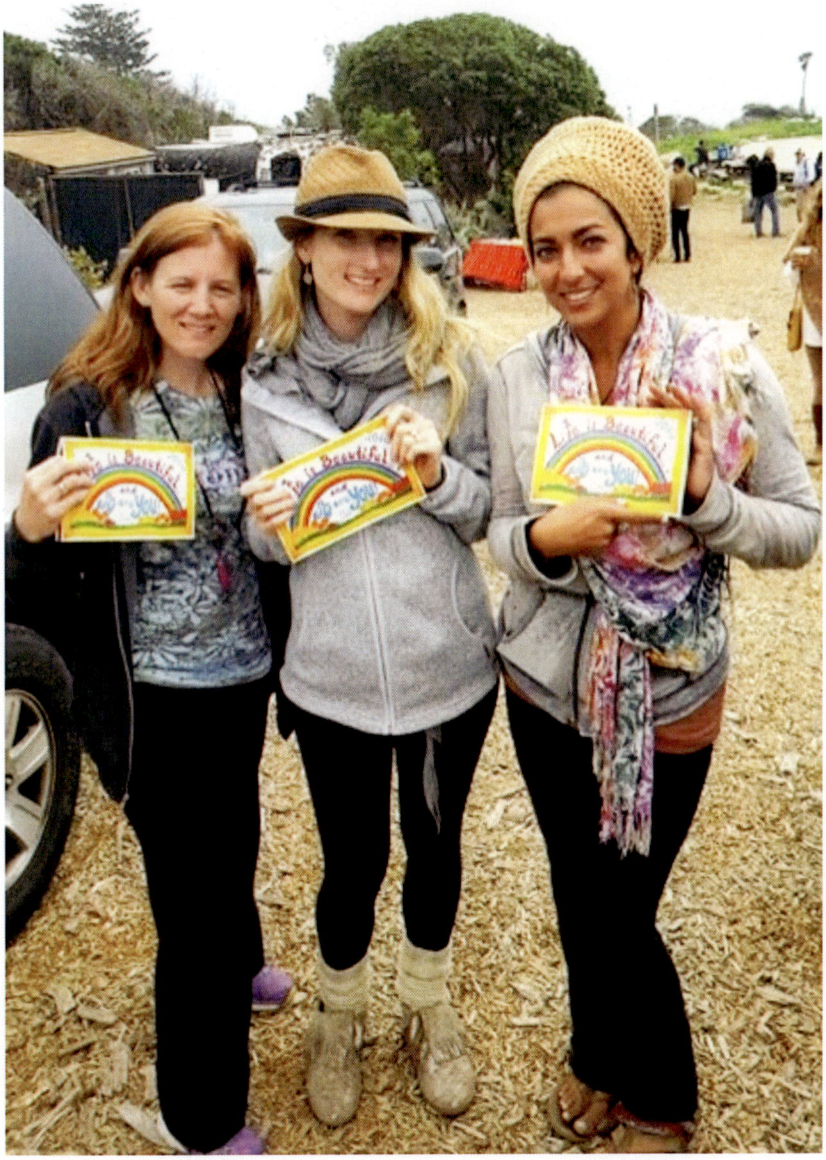

Yogi Goddesses @ Chumash Village

♥Green Salad

Serves: 4
Time: 15 minutes

1 head Leafy Green Lettuce
½ Cucumber. Sliced thinly into rounds
½ Beet, shredded in food processor
3 Carrots, shredded in food processor
1 tomato, cut into bite-size "chunks"
½ container Sunflower sprouts

1) Wash + break apart/ cut lettuce, into bite-size pieces. Arrange lettuce in a circular salad bowl. Shred carrots + beets. Cut cucumber + tomato.
2) Decorate with cucumber slices, sunflower sprouts, tomato, carrot + beets in a mandala around the edges of the bowl.
3) Enjoy with Cashew Ranch, Tahini or other dressing! Simple + Easy!

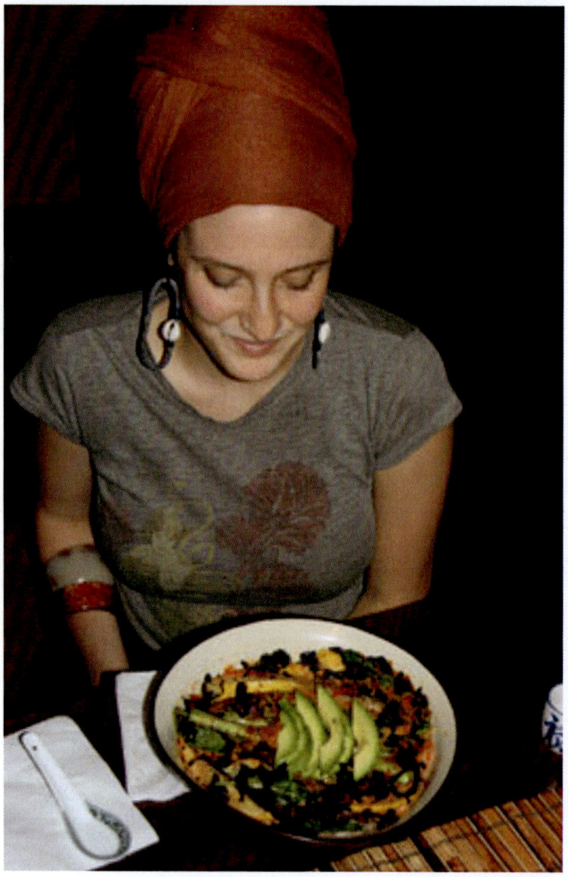

More Breakfast Delights

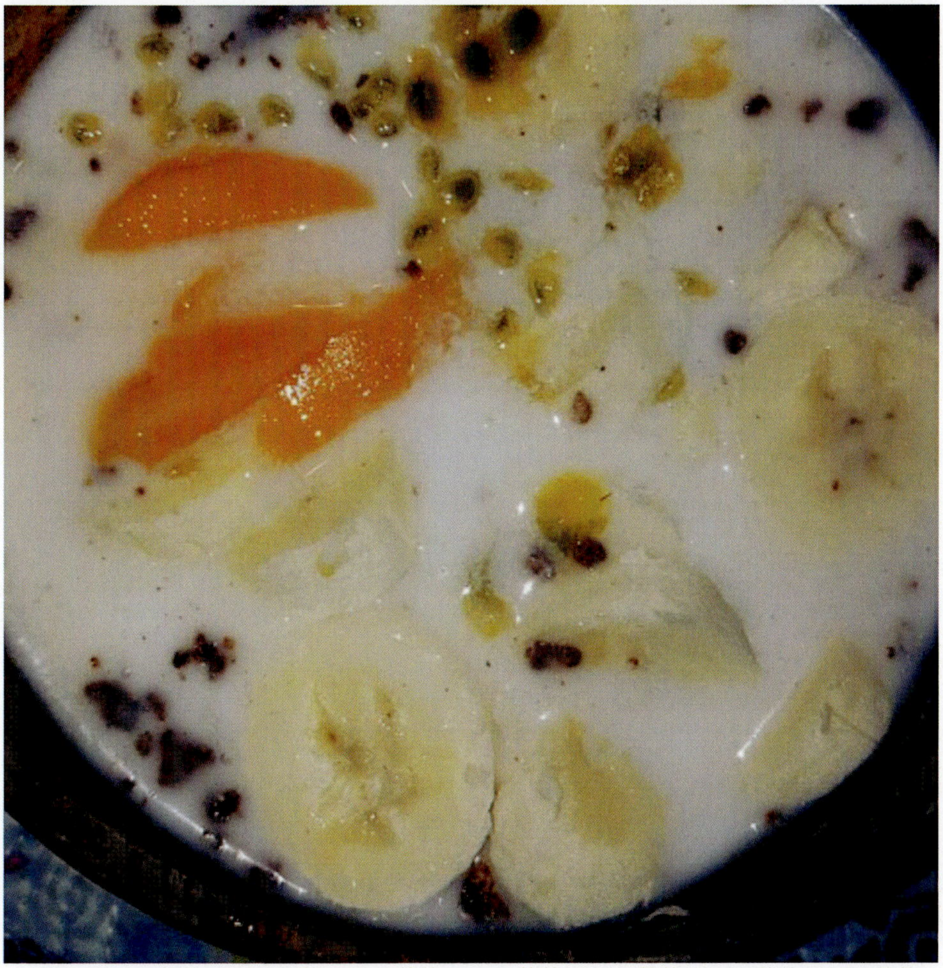

Organic non-GMO Grits

Serves: 6
Time: 35 minutes

This recipe is so simple + easy, but it is delicious! Growing up in Texas from age one to six, we ate grits! When I moved to the South in my twenties, I learned that grits were popular, as the corn was locally grown, and I started eating grits again! When I worked at The Local Farmstand, we sold locally grown corn grits! This recipe reminds me of that time. I LOVE grits!

4 c filtered water
1 c organic non-GMO corn grits
1 tsp sea salt
2 T coconut oil

1) In a pot, heat water to boil w/ sea salt.
2) When water is boiling, gradually stir in grits. Bring heat to low + simmer, stirring frequently, to prevent clumps, for 15 minutes, or until cooked!
3) When grits are done, add coconut oil for "buttery" taste. Yum Yum! Southern comfort!

♥∆Raw Vegan Sausages: A Debra Classic

Serves: 8
Time: 30 minutes prep, 4 hours dehydration (requires overnight soaking of sunflower seeds + dates)

Did you know the word "sau-sage" comes from the spice "sage?" It's true! The taste of "sausage" is really in the spices. Here's my old joke from a decade ago, when I was dating women + this recipe was born.

Q: Why are so many lesbians vegetarian?
A: Because they love that Fake Meat!!!

(Oh, silly, silly! ;))

4 c soaked sunflower seeds
½ c soaked dates
½ c yellow onion
3 T sage powder
1 tsp cayenne pepper
1 T fennel seeds
1 t sea salt
filtered water

1) Soak sunflower seeds overnight, rinse + drain. Soak dates overnight too!
2) Food process everything in this order: 1) onion 2) sunflower seeds 3) dates 4) everything else 5) filtered water, just enough to turn the mix.
3) Shape into dehydrator sheets. Dehydrate @ about 105 degrees.
4) Flip when solid enough (usually about 3 hours). Dry for another hour. They should be solid on the outside, yet soft on the inside. And darken on the outside too! ;)
5) Yum Yum! These take a minute to dehydrate, but are SOO worth it!

"Leftover" Dessert Favorites

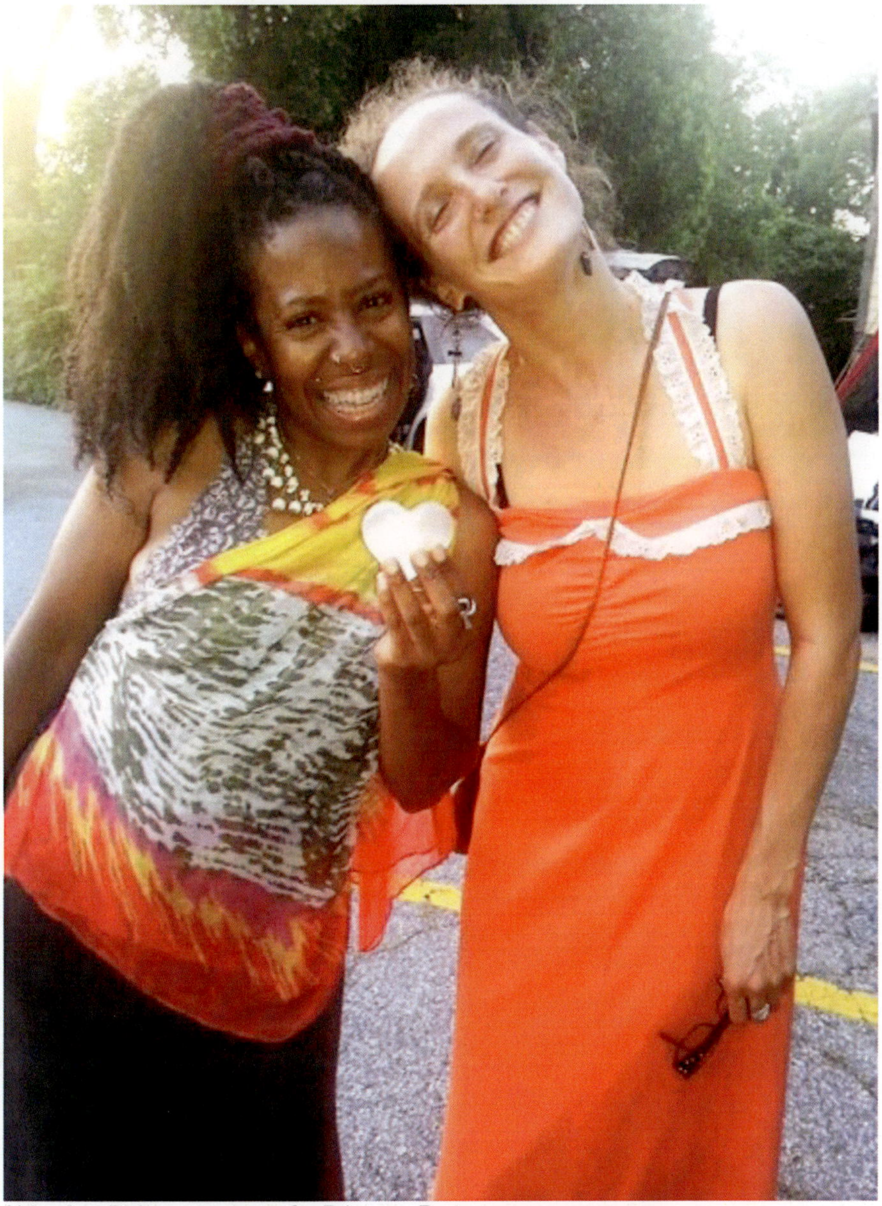

Ahl-vah + Debra, creators of a Princess Party, many moons ago…

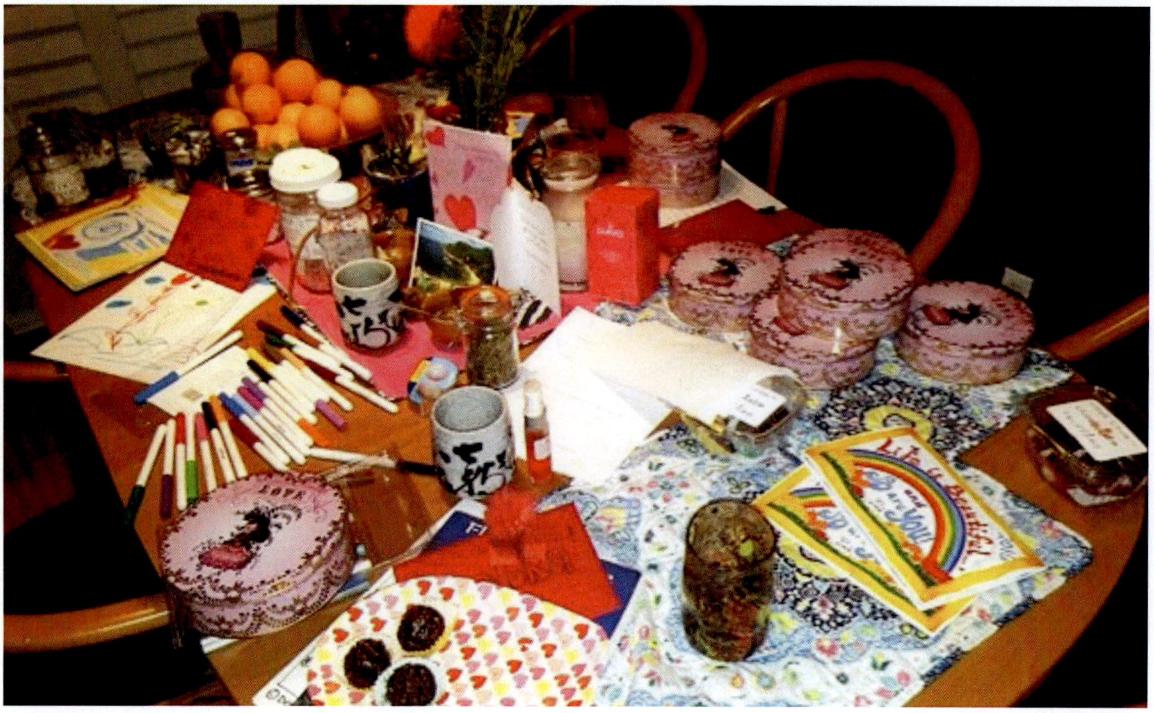
Life is Beautiful

ΔSweet Coconut Rice w/ Seasonal Fruit
Serves: 6
Time: 15 minutes (not including cooking rice, in which case, 1 hour ;) + would also require overnight soaking of rice)

2 c Brown Rice, cooked
2/3 can coconut milk
4 T raw local honey
1 ripe mango, sliced
1 tsp brown sesame seeds (optional)
pinch sea salt
½ tsp vanilla

1) This recipe works great with plain leftover brown rice, if you're looking for something fun to do with it! The idea is you make your rice, then you get to use it for a lot of things! If using freshly cooked Rice, please soak rice overnight, then drain, rinse, + cook!
2) Blend coconut milk, local honey, sea salt + vanilla. Then pour over cool, cooked brown rice.
3) Stir together till well blended, sweet + yummy. Add sweetener/ coconut milk if needed.
4) Top with mango slices! You can also sprinkle a few brown sesame seeds, for decoration!

ΔBlack Bean Brownies – Gluten-Free, Sugar-Free, Vegan + Delicious!
Serves: 12
Time: 45 minutes (requires overnight soaking of black beans, if leftover beans are not used ;))

1 ½ c black beans, cooked
2 T raw cacao powder
½ c gluten-free rolled oats
¼ tsp sea salt
½ c Grade B maple syrup
¼ c coconut oil
2 tsp vanilla extract
½ tsp baking powder
½ c chocolate chips or walnuts! (Optional! ;))

1) Use leftover black beans, or soak black beans overnight, rinse, drain + cook!
2) In food processor, process oats. When chopped fine, add black beans to food processor. When this is smooth, add all other ingredients, with the exception of chocolate chips.
3) Transfer batter to a mixing bowl + fold in chocolate chips, walnuts, or other fun ingredients!
4) Grease a glass baking pan with coconut oil + pour batter in.
5) Bake at 350 degrees for 20 minutes. Or until fork comes out clean. ;)
6) Cool + cut into squares! Enjoy! So healthy + delicious!! ;)

Secret Special Desserts

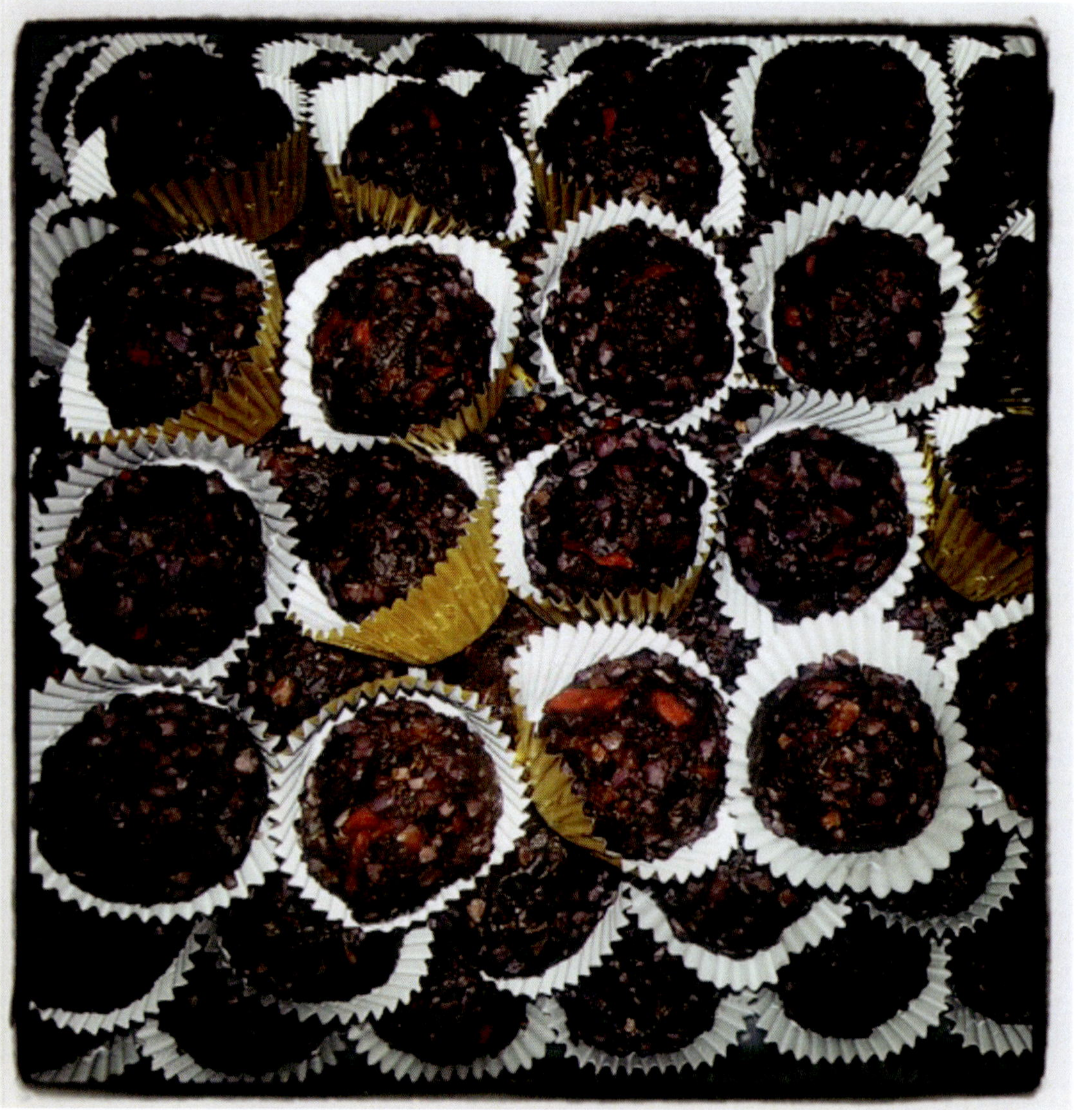

Cacao Elixir Tea Drink

Serves: 8
Time: 40 minutes (including steep time)

This recipe is treasured + often requested! I thought twice about sharing it here, but I'm doing it! This is a great coffee alternative, for its warmth + cacao energy. It has a silky, peaceful, blissful, comforting, uplifting vibe. Enjoy at any time of day. ;)

5 Spring Dragon tea bags (by Ron Teeguarden)
¼ c cacao butter
1/3 c cacao powder
1/3 c Grade B maple syrup
1 t vanilla extract
¼ t sea salt
1 t chlorella
6-8 cups filtered water

1) Boil filtered water. When boiling, turn off heat, + steep teabags. Steep for 30 minutes or more, for best results.
2) Pour warm tea in the blender/ Vitamix, + add all other ingredients. Blend carefully, placing a thick towel or potholder over the top of the blender, so hot water does not splash/ or drip out.
3) Pour into a beautiful mug + enjoy. Pass around at a tea party. Share with a friend.

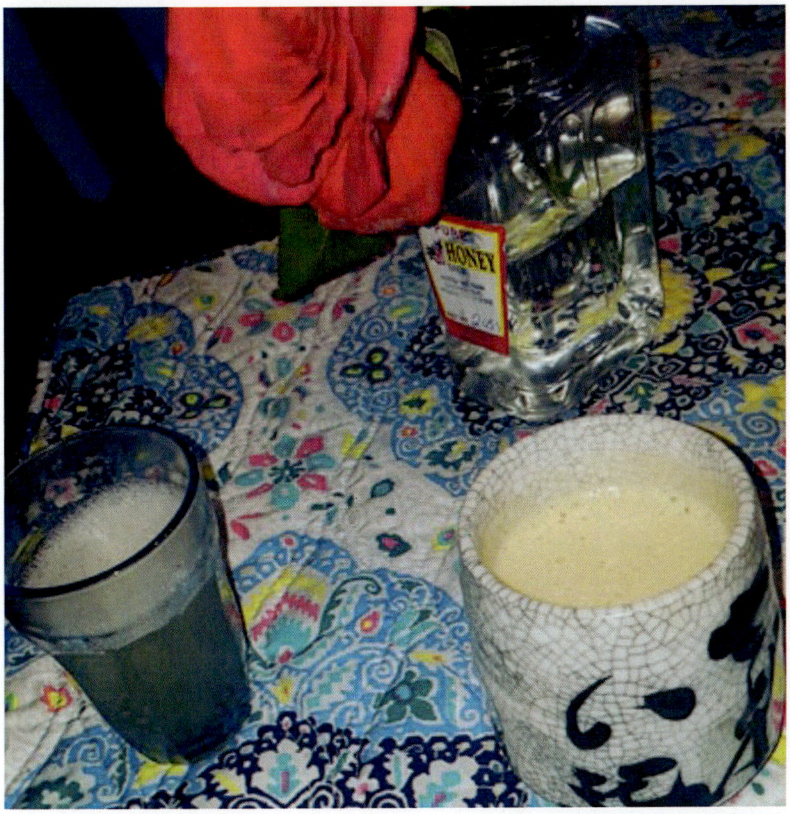

♥Hot Love Chocolate Truffles™

Debra's organic cuisine is an extraordinary experience of nutritional ecstasy, whether for a catered meal or a Hot Love [Chocolate] Truffle - this is passionate, life-giving food!" – Shiva Rea

(Did you really think I was going to give you the Hot Love Chocolate Truffle™ recipe?!! ;) Nope! That one is off limits! It's my billion-dollar, most-requested item! ;)) Hot Love Chocolate Truffles™ are Best of Raw Award-Winning!

But you can learn more: DebraMazer.com

While you're there, sign up for Love + Inspiration Notes – they're FREE! And you'll get another e-book for FREE too! It's called Morning Rituals Playbook: 25 Ideas to Create Peace + Balance in Your Life.

I'm a Life Coach too! And Holistic Life Coach! I have more Recipe Books + Spiritual Books for your reading + learning adventure. Come allow yourself to be supported as you transform into the Butterfly that you are! Into your most Wildly Creative, Vibrant, + Thriving Life!

Find out more: DebraMazer.com

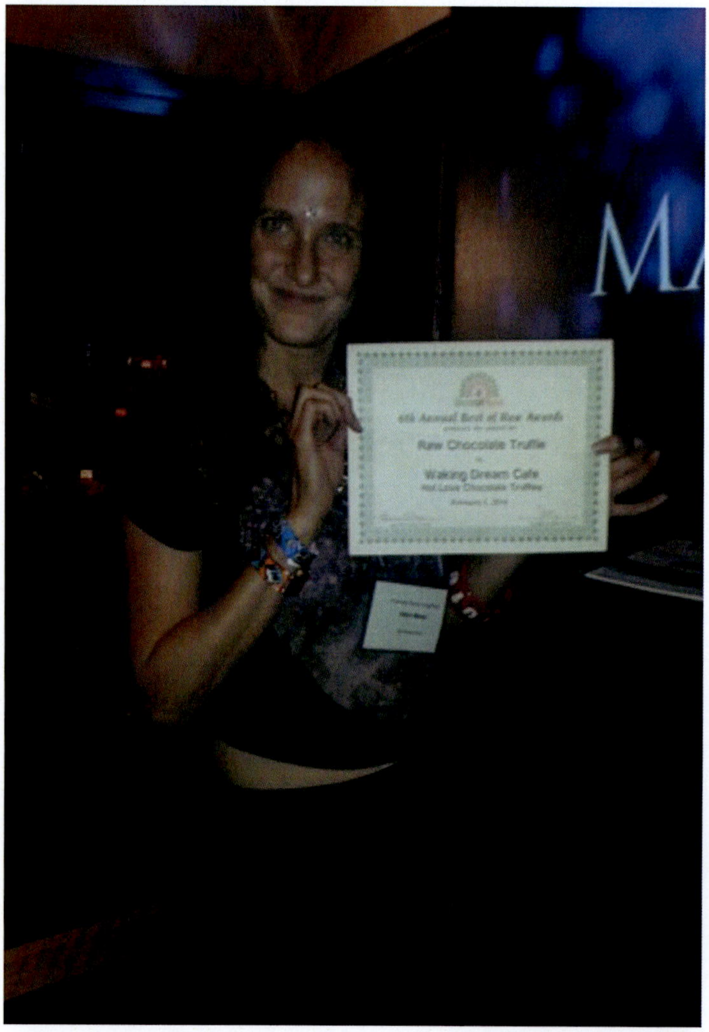

About the Author:

"Check out Debra Jill Mazer! I want to play with her, she seems awesome!" – Alicia Silverstone, Actress

"I love Debra's beautiful spirit and her delicious recipes! She's a kind, compassionate, sparkly, talented soul." – Kris Carr, NY Times Bestselling Author, Crazy Sexy Kitchen

You might know Debra as a Spiritual Author, Life Coach + Winner of the Best of Raw Awards. But really, she's a Thought Leader, Wise Teacher, + Prayer Warrior.

Debra Mazer is *magna cum laude* graduate of Brandeis University, with a B.A. in Sociology + Women's Studies Program Member. She graduated high school with a 4.0 + won the Math Award several times. ;)

Debra Mazer is author of the acclaimed Open-Eyed Heart-Wide Haggadah, New Raw, Little Red Recipes, My Life in Hair (out of print), and Retreat Recipes for Yoga Lovers.

She is a trained + Certified Life Coach through LifeWorks School of Coaching in Atlanta, and a Certified Holistic Health Coach through the Institute for Integrative Nutrition in NYC.

Winner of The Best of Raw Awards for her Hot Love Chocolate Truffles™, she has appeared on Today.com, Huffington Post, Alicia Silverstone's TheKindLife.com, KrisCarr.com, and more.

Debra is a graduate of the Living Foods Institute in Atlanta, having served as their Kitchen Director + Lead Instructor in 2005, 2008.

As a Retreat Chef, she has worked under David Wolfe, Elaina Love, Melissa Mango + Jackie Graff. Her business, Vibrance, appeared as a 3-page cover in the Atlanta-Journal Constitution, and she catered a private dinner for Kris Carr, pre-Oprah days.

It has been her joy + honor to cater for Shiva Rea's Yoga Teacher Trainings/ Retreats in California.

She's currently working on her Dream Autobiography Memoir Book, another Recipe Book, new Coaching Programs, Interview Series + more!

Debra dreams of owning an Amethyst Biomat + Infrared Sauna, traveling to Bali, + flying on a private jet w/ Oprah, Michelle Obama, Barack, + Richard Branson! (I mean, why not put the energy out there?!) She loves trampolines + her favorite place on earth is Harbin Hot Springs.

Check out DebraMazer.com + Receive a FREE copy of her e-book, Morning Rituals Playbook, to spice up your life + break out of the box!

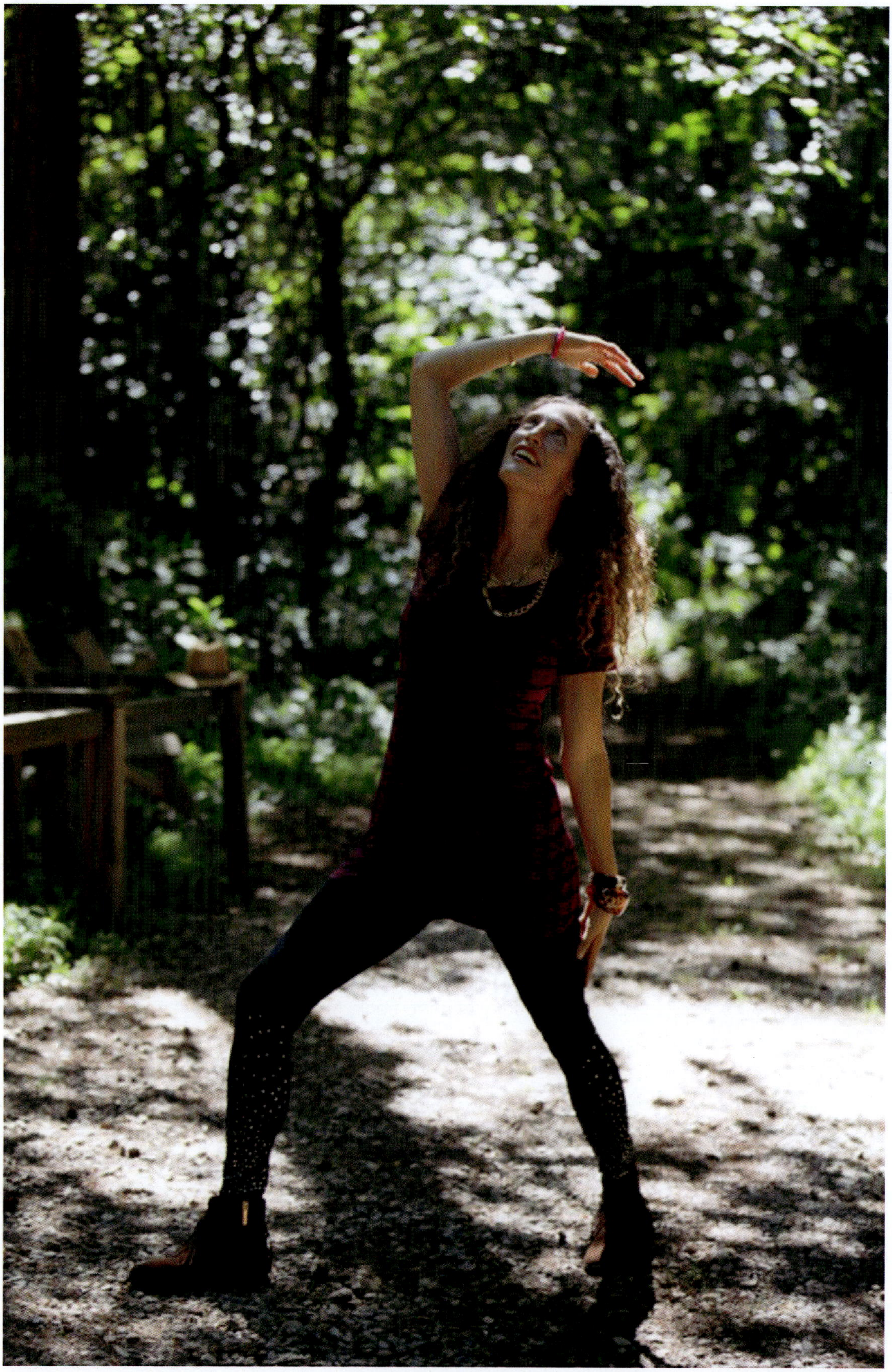

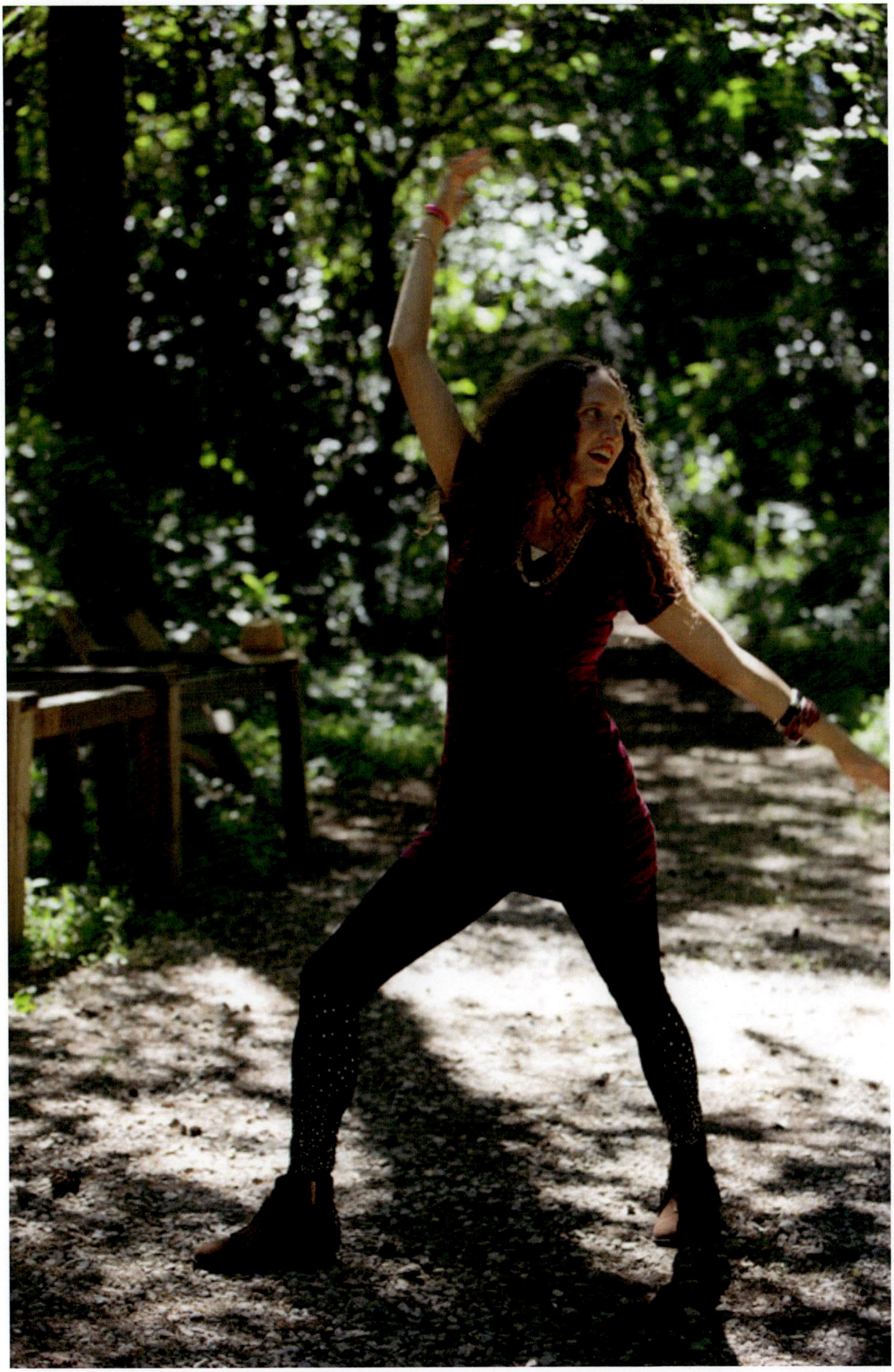

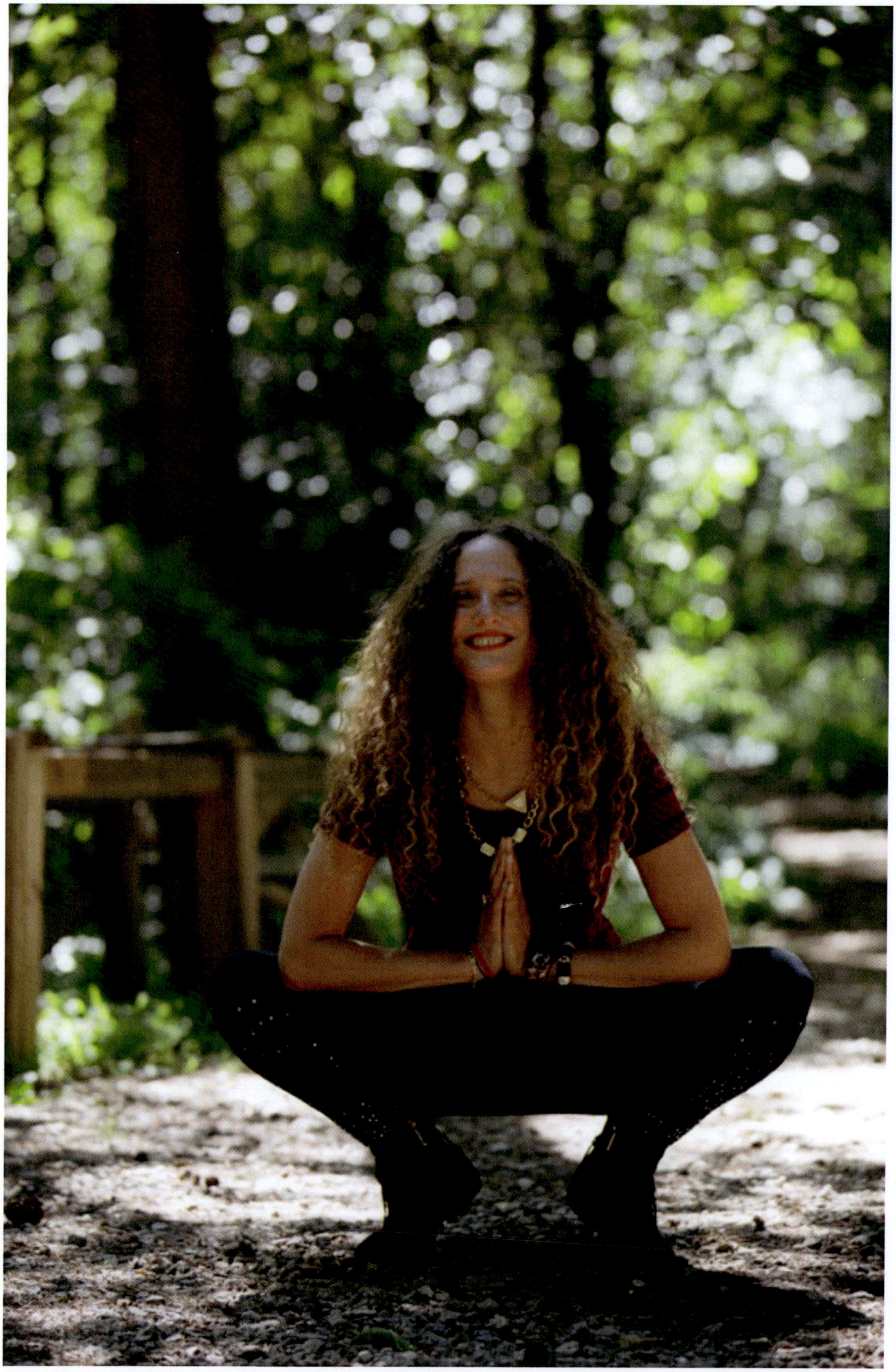